CZECHOSLOVAK ACADEMY OF SCIENCES

# The Morphology
# and Pathogenicity
# of the Bladder Worms

*Cysticercus cellulosae* and *Cysticercus bovis*

# CZECHOSLOVAK ACADEMY OF SCIENCES

*Scientific Editor Academician Otto Jírovec*
*Scientific Adviser Prof. Dr. Josef Vaněk*
*Language Editor Eva Kalinová*

# The Morphology and Pathogenicity of the Bladder Worms

*Cysticercus cellulosae* and *Cysticercus bovis*

JAROSLAV ŠLAIS

1970

Springer-Verlag
Berlin Heidelberg GmbH

ACADEMIA

*Publishing House of the*
*Czechoslovak Academy of Sciences, Prague*

ISBN 978-90-6193-250-5      ISBN 978-94-011-6466-5 (eBook)
DOI 10.1007/978-94-011-6466-5

# Contents

# Introduction

The larval stage of taeniid cestodes, called the cysticercus, develops in the intermediate host from the oncosphere. The infection caused by cysticerci is called cysticercosis. Man is the only definitive host of two adult cestode species. One of them is the cestode *Taenia solium* Linné, 1758. Its larva is called *Cysticercus cellulosae* developing mostly in the muscles of swine. The other is *Taeniarhynchus saginatus* Goeze, 1782 and its larva *Cysticercus bovis* (*C. inermis*) develops in the muscles of cattle. Man can carry a cysticercus being its intermediate host, and suffer from cysticercosis.

Because cysticerci are localized in the muscles of livestock, various measures have to be taken to prevent an infection of man with the adult cestode. These include a very strict inspection of the carcasses at the abattoir, a special treatment of infected meat or a certificate declaring it unfit for human consumption. The incidence of human tapeworms, being still relatively high in the population, can be controlled successfully only by a comprehensive programme of eradication of muscle cysticercosis. There is no exact information available on fundamental processes in the biology of the cysticercus such as its development, its initial growth in the muscles, its metabolism, the length of its life, the reaction of the host, the possibility of spontaneous healing. Such knowledge is not only of theoretical importance, but indispensable for successful control of the parasites and for the serological diagnosis of cysticercosis.

The present study, based on the results of the author's 10-year-investigation, is an attempt to solve fundamental questions of the morphology, morphogenesis, histochemistry and pathogenicity of the two cysticerci, which are most important for man. This comprehensive account may be used as a basis for further research on the physiology and immunology of these parasites and for their successful control.

Our studies were based on 9 observations of cerebral cysticercosis or generalized cysticercosis of man and on 3 observations of the racemose form of cerebral cysticercosis. Histological examinations were performed on 24 cysticerci from a massive cysticercosis of the brain leading to the sudden death of the patient. Therefore, we obtained from this material only the younger and normal developmental stages of the parasite. In the study of generalized cysticercosis we examined 12 parasites from the cerebellum and the diaphragm, 13 cysticerci from the brain, the heart and the skeletal muscles. We examined 22 morphologically well preserved parasites from a case of protracted cysticercosis with a high incidence of parasites in the meninges and the brain. In this

Table 1.

Survey of clinical data relevant to the material from cysticercosis of man

| Material no. | Age in years | Sex | Type of cysticercosis | Number and state of cysticerci | Origin of material |
|---|---|---|---|---|---|
| 1 | 50 | m | Multiple cysticercosis of the meninges and the cortex; 3 scars with remnants of the parasite in the brain matter | 31 cysticerci ranging from fully developed to minute remnants in the scars | Šikl's Dept. of Pathol., Medical Faculty, Plzeň no. biop. 11871—2/53 (ŠLAIS 1965) |
| 2 | 52 | f | solitary cysticercus in meninges | parasitic remnants in the connective tissue scar | do. no. biop. 8333—4/57 (ŠLAIS 1965) |
| 3 | 76 | f | multiple muscle cysticercosis of the thorax and the arm | numerous parasites in the muscles, one in the heart, one in the brain. All parasites in connective tissue scars at an advanced stage of resorption | do. autopsy no. 297/63 (ŠLAIS 1965) |
| 4 | 77 | f | multiple cysticercosis of meninges and cortex | developed parasites, reaction ranging from minimal to fibrous encapsulation | Ist Dept. of Pathol., Medical Faculty, Prague, autopsy no. 1009/36 |
| 5 | 55 | f | solitary focus in basal brain ganglia | cysticercus at advanced stage of resorption | do. autopsy no. 163/53 |
| 6 | Museum material no. 237/III— 5151 | | extensive and diffuse cerebral cysticercosis | young stages with marked inflammatory reaction — up to 30 cysticerci to 50 ccm of brain tissue | IInd Dept. of Pathol., Medical Faculty, Prague |

| Material no. | Age in years | Sex | Type of cysticercosis | Number and state of cysticerci | Origin of material |
|---|---|---|---|---|---|
| 7 | 29 Museum material no. 249 | f | multiple cysticercosis of meninges and brain | parasites at a stage of advanced resorption, one cysticercus lying freely in the 4th ventricle | do. (HAMMER 1889) |
| 8 | Museum material no. 264/III 5777 | | multiple cysticercosis of meninges and brain | completely developed cysticerci, several degenerated cysts | do |
| 9 | — | m | generalized cysticercosis | numerous parasites with signs of dystrophy in the cerebellum and the diaphragm | Dept. of Pathol., Haiphong hospital |
| 10 | 54 | f | racemose cysticercus | an originally large cysticercus in sulcus corporis callosi; its bladder continued to grow at the base of the brain | Ist Dept. of Pathol., Medical Faculty, Prague, autopsy no. 1119/64 (ŠLAIS, KALUŠ 1967) |
| 11 | 27 | m | racemose cysticercus | tumorous formation of the size of an egg in the temporo-parietal brain region formed by the proliferating bladders of the parasite | do. biopsy no. 2302/47 |
| 12 | 71 | f | racemose cysticercus | grapelike cystic formations of parasitic bladders in the meninges on the base of the brain | do. autopsy no 1344/49 (KARPÍŠEK, VALACH 1952) |

observation, in a similar cysticercosis obtained from a museum collection and also in some solitary findings we examined 29 shrivelled and necrotic cysts or their calcified remnants. Only in 5 cases, which were at an advanced stage of resorption, were we unable to identify the morphology of the parasite. Altogether our morphological studies were performed on 95 parasites from cysticercosis of man. In addition we studied also the complicated formations of the racemose cysticercus. By using a special method it was possible to reconstruct and establish the morphology of the parasites even in necrotic, calcified cysts or in cysts with partly resorbed contents. Basic information on the material used is given in table 1; clinical histories can be found in a previous paper (ŠLAIS 1965, ŠLAIS and KALUŠ 1967).

For comparison we studied *C. cellulosae* from a massive infestation of the musculature of swine. Partial or complete series of histological sections were made from 37 parasites, of which 30 cysticerci were embedded in paraffin along with the surrounding tissue. With the same method we examined 110 cysts from a cysticercosis of the skeletal muscles and the heart of cattle. In addition to histological procedures, 640 *C. bovis* were removed from their enclosing connective tissue to be observed in saline solution and to assess their viability. Their evagination was accomplished mechanically by pressure or occurred spontaneously in a saline solution. After evagination the cysticerci were fixed and some of them were cut into series of histological sections. In another 140 cysts it was not possible to identify the morphologically preserved remnants of the parasite macroscopically. The material for studies on *C. cellulosae* and *C. bovis* was obtained from the Prague abattoir. The process of evagination was observed experimentally in viable *C. pisiformis*, removed from cysts on the omentum of rabbits (50 larvae). We examined also material consisting of *C. crassiceps* from the abdominal cavity of *Microtus arvalis*, and of *C. tenuicollis* from the abdominal cavity of an elk from the Zoological Garden of Prague.

The development of *C. cellulosae* was traced in a cerebral cysticercosis of man from larvae of 1 mm in diameter to necrotic and decayed larvae; in addition from larvae of 2 mm in diameter up to the typical cysticerci in a muscle cysticercosis of swine. *C. bovis* was found at the stage of a mother bladder, measuring 0·7 and 1·5 mm in diameter. Moreover we studied larvae terminating their development and also their very aged to necrotic forms in a muscle cysticercosis of cattle. The morphogenesis of the mother bladder was studied in *C. tenuicollis* during experimental and natural infection. The complete development from the mother bladder to the very old form was encountered in *C. crassiceps*.

The microscopic structure of the bladder-wall of *C. cellulosae* was studied in viable and dead, fully developed cysticerci in a brain cysticercosis of man and also in larvae in a muscle cysticercosis of swine. The bladder of *Coenurus cerebralis* was examined in material from a museum collection and in other experimental material (Parasitological Department of the Zoological Institute, Prague; Institute of Helminthology (VIGIZ), Moscow; Kazakh'Scientific Veterinary Institute, Alma Ata; Parasitological Laboratory, Dzhambul.

# Histological methods

Fresh material was fixed with Schaffer's fluid or in 10% formol; the material from the museum collection was in formol, alcohol or in Kaiserling's fluid. Sometimes, long storage had made the identification of calcium by Kossa's method impossible. However, the staining properties of material stored for some tens of years in alcohol were not affected. We embedded most of the cysts in paraffin, but especially for the identification of the number of hooks and their shape, we mounted some after a fine dissection in Canada balsam. Also small pieces of the bladder wall were stained with iron haematoxylin after Weigert or as membranes in the procedure after Jasvoin and then mounted on slides. These were examined by phase contrast microscope.

Necrotic and calcified material, was decalcified, if necessary, in 5% trichloracidic acid, perfectly dehydrated and infiltrated with very hard paraffin to obtain the most complete series of histological sections possible. Such are generally needed for the identification of these formations. Their content is not homogeneous and the exudate component tends to become brittle and to chip off after being embedded in paraffin. It is also difficult to cut the hard and chalklike crumbling content of the cyst owing to its different hardness compared with that of the surrounding tissue. The contents of the cyst can be prevented from crumbling or chipping off during cutting by breathing on the surface of the paraffin block before each cut to warm it. Should the paraffin not be hard enough it is necessary to cool the surface of the block with a piece of ice before cutting. This occurs especially when the room temperature is too high. Important also is the thickness of the section which should not exceed 4—6 µm because thicker sections generally tend to break. A complete extension of the section can be achieved only by the help of very hot water. A perfect adherence of the sections to the slides can be obtained by immediately placing them with the fully extended sections for 1/2 h into the incubator at 58 °C and then continuing to dry them at 40 °C.

The most important method for the staining of the sections is the regressive modification of Giemsa's method: paraffin-free sections are subjected to staining for 24 h in a solution (0·2 ml stock-solution diluted in 10 ml distilled water), then rinsed in distilled water and, under microscopic control, differentiated with 1% acetic acid. After rapid rinsing in several changes of acetone and acetone–xylol, the slides are transferred into xylol and mounted in Caedax or neutral Canada balsam. In this way the hooks of the cestodes, the other cuticular formations of the parasites and the proteinic skeletons of the calcareous corpuscles are coloured blue. A certain differentiation of the necrotic structures can be obtained with Weigert-van Gieson's method. Especially suitable is Goldner's method, which stains red also the hooks of the cestodes and parts of the cuticular formations. The most suitable method for demonstrating the remnants of necrotic and disintegrating structures of the cysticercus is Gomori's technique for reticular fibres, this being successful even in cases, in which with the haematoxylin-eosin the contents appear almost homogeneous. It requires, however, a perfect adherence of the section to the slide to prevent silver precipitation on uneven parts and in fine fissures. Another suitable method is Mallory's phosphotungstic haematoxylin. The degree of autolysis of the parasite's tissues was determined by the loss of staining power of the cell nuclei with Feulgen's reaction. The microscopic anatomy of the necrotic cysticerci could be clearly demonstrated with Goldner's staining and Gomori's technique. It was mostly possible to make reconstructions of these remnants of the parasites and to confirm the morphological development of the cysticercus during the last phase of its survival in the host's tissue. In addition to other standard histological and cytological methods we used also techniques for the identification of Ca, Fe, pigments, neuroglia, nervous fibres, the DNA and lipids. Polysaccharides were detected with the following methods: PAS with acetylation, desacetylation and the saliva test, Hale's method in Müller's modification, Mowry's technique using only colloidal iron on the control slides and in combination with the PAS reaction; alcian blue (AB) with neutral red by Steedman's technique and in a solution of sulphuric acid; metachromasy was tested with thionine, toluidine blue at a different pH and with the Pearse's MBET (methylene blue extinction test). Proteins were detected histologically with Millon's reaction, the DMAB method after Adams, Sakaguchi's technique for arginine, DDD (2,2-dihydroxy-6,6-dinaphthylsulphite) method for the detection of SH-groups and the PFAS, PAA-AF and PFA-AB method (performic acid-Schiff, peracetic acid-aldehyde fuchsin and performic acid — alcian blue techniques).

# Morphology of the egg and the oncosphere of taeniids

The cestodes *T. solium* and *Trh.* (= *Taeniarhynchus*) *saginatus* are transmitted by man, the definitive host. The gravid segments expelled with the faeces are just containers of a great number of eggs. The embryonated eggs are released and become a source of infection for the intermediate host. Nowadays, *T. solium* has almost disappeared from Western and Eastern Europe, pigs being bred in modern pigsties without free runs; on the contrary, the incidence of *Trh. saginatus* is still quite high, which may be due to the way in which cattle are kept, but is mainly due to the manuring of pastures with sewage. This causes an uneven incidence of cysticerci in meat, it being sometimes too low to be noticed in the inspection of the carcasses. Therefore, when describing the egg and the oncosphere, attention has been given mainly to *Trh. saginatus* (Fig. 1).

The eggs in the early, gravid segments are surrounded with a cytoplasmic layer (outer envelope). This is followed by a thick, striated embryophore. The cytoplasmic layer is easily lost and, in the gravid segments, most of the oncospheres remain covered with the embryophore. The diameter of such eggs is 55—75 µm by 40—55 µm. The embryophore is 0·03—0·04 mm thick.

PAVLOVA (1963) distinguished two layers in the embryophore of *Trh. saginatus*: a) the peripheral-granular layer; b) the inner, radially striated layer. A similar structure was observed in *Taenia serrata* (JANICKI 1907). This radial striation is caused by elongate blocks joined by a cement substance. According to LEE et al. (1959), these embryophoric blocks are formed by a coalescence of the aggregates of granules developing gradually from the fine, granular layer which covers the oncosphere. This primary layer is of a cellular, syncytial nature.

Recent studies indicate that the embryophore consists of four layers. The outer one, a colourless, gelatinous membrane is followed by a proteinic layer, which is relatively thick, grayish-yellow to brown, radially striated. The second proteinic layer is thin with a dark-yellow outline. The innermost layer covering directly the oncosphere is of a lipoid nature. Pepsin and trypsin dissolve the embryophore which, however, is not affected by erepsin. The three outer layers are permeable to water, solutions of salts and to alcohol (up to 80%). The innermost layer is impermeable to these solutions, but can be dissolved in chloroform and ether.

The inner surface of the embryophore of *Trh. saginatus* stains differently with various histological methods. The outer, thick surface is highly refractile and, therefore, it was impossible to reveal by histochemical methods the presence of a membrane covering the embryophore. The yellow colour observed in the histological sections seems to be caused rather by high refraction than by a real colour. The embryophore is formed by thick rods of the basic substance arranged radially towards the centre of the egg and joined by a cement substance of different chemical properties. In its outermost part in up to half of its width we observed coarser granules. The staining properties of all these structures are shown in table 2.

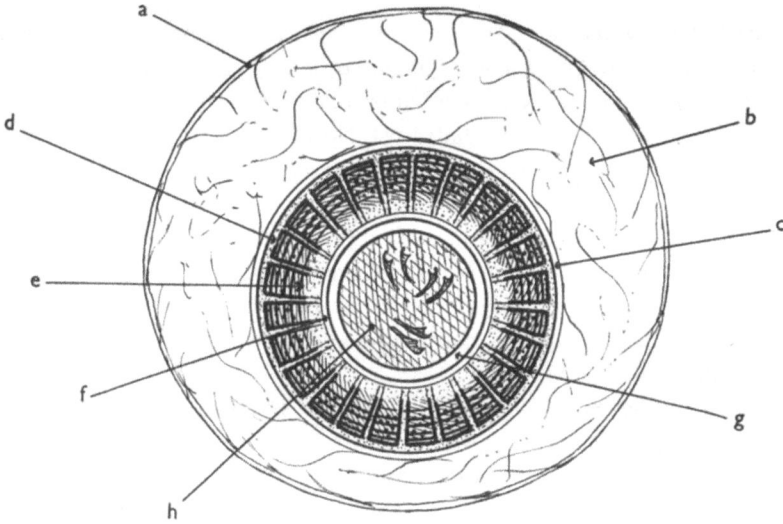

Fig. 1. Schematic illustration of the morphology of the egg of *Taeniarhynchus saginatus*. Outer envelope = a — capsule; b — vitelline layer; c — outermost cover of the embryophore (remnant of the vitelline layer after the loss of the outer envelopes); d — outermost layer of the embryophore; e — embryophoric blocks; f — innermost layer of the embryophore; g — oncospheral membrane; h — oncosphere.

The electron microscope revealed structural details in the egg membranes. The first exhaustive histological description was given by SKVORTSOV (1942). MORSETH (1965) detected the presence of an outermost, thin layer on the surface of the embryophore. He noticed that the embryophoric blocks begin to form beneath the outer membrane increasing in length towards the embryo. The high refraction of the granules in the outer, embryophoric zone has been of interest even to earlier investigators (LEUCKART 1881—1887, BENEDEN 1881, SAINT-REMY 1901, JANICKI 1907). According to Morseth, these are, in fact, lacunae in the substance of the blocks in which the circular bodies persist. These are the focal points around which the dense, embryophoric block substance is deposited while the embryophore develops. PAVLOVA'S concept (1965) that the peripheral, granular structure in the embryophore

## Table 2.

Results of some histological and histochemical methods in studies of the embryophore of the eggs of *Taeniarhynchus saginatus*

| Methods | Embryophore | | | |
|---|---|---|---|---|
| | Blocks | Cement substance | Granulation of the outer layers of the embryophore | Inner surface of embryophore |
| Haematoxylin-eosin | feebly rose coloured | feebly red | 0 | brilliant red |
| van Gieson | intense yellow | reddish | 0 | red |
| Trichrome after Masson | natural colour | reddish | 0 | red |
| Trichrome after Goldner | feebly orange | reddish | 0 | red in some eggs |
| Mallory's phosphotungstic haematoxylin | brownish-violet | 0 | intense bluish-violet | 0 |
| Giemsa | blue | dark blue | mostly undifferentiated, sometimes dark blue | 0 |
| Ziehl-Neelsen | intense red-violet | indistinguishable from the blocks | indistinguishable | 0 |
| Best | natural colour | 0 | 0 | red |
| PAS | natural colour | 0 | 0 | 0 |
| Hale-PAS | natural colour | 0 | 0 | 0 |
| Hale | intense yellow | reddish | 0 | reddish |
| PAA-AF | feebly coloured | red-violet | 0 | feebly coloured |

Table 2.

| PFA-AB | natural colour | 0 | sometimes indicated by refraction | 0 |
|---|---|---|---|---|
| AB, pH 0·2 | natural colour | 0 | 0 | 0 |
| Adams'reaction | natural colour | 0 | 0 | 0 |
| Millon | ++++ | 0 | 0 | 0 |
| ninhydrin-Schiff | natural colour | 0 | 0 | 0 |
| arginine | natural colour | 0 | 0 | 0 |

originates from the direct secretion of the embryo is, therefore, not correct. The nature of the circular bodies could not be revealed even under the electron microscope.*
They stain only with Mallory's phosphotungstic haematoxylin, while the cement substance between the blocks does not stain with this but with other histological methods. Electron microscopy revealed a communication between the lacunae of the embryophore and the cement substance between the blocks. This substance passes into the inner layer of the embryophore in which the blocks terminate. This layer is of granular nature being a remnant of the embryophoric cells secreting the blocks. The inner layer is of variable thickness, lined with a very delicate, basal membrane. Beneath it lies the oncospheral membrane and the limiting membrane covering the embryo. The exceptional resistance of the embryophore and its morphological and staining properties have greatly attracted earlier investigators. As with the cestode hooks, the embryophore was considered also to consist of chitin although no proof was given. Its bright-yellow staining with picric acid, similar to that of the egg capsules in turbellarians, trematodes and pseudophyllidean cestodes suggests the presence of a protein. In the latter groups the substance of the egg capsules was identified as a sclerotin, i.e. a quinone-tanned protein. This capsule, however, is not homologous with the embryophore of the cyclophyllideans, but with their early capsule (SMYTH and CLEGG 1959, RYBICKA 1966). We found that the embryophoric blocks give

---

*) According to M. L. NIELAND (J. Parasit. 54 : 957—969, 1968), the circular bodies appear, in *Hydatigera* (*T.*) *taeniaeformis*, to be mitochondria which in the initial stages of embryophore formation do not seem to be the focal points for deposition of the block substance. Possibly they are involved in the synthesis or maintenance of integrity of the cement substance between the blocks.

a highly positive reaction for tyrosin. JOHRI (1957) using bromphenol blue and PFAS-reaction for SS-groups, indicated the presence of a "keratin" type of protein. Also MORSETH (1966) obtained positive results with PFAS, studying the embryophore also by the use of chromatography, infrared spectroscopy and nitrogen and sulphur determination. He concluded that a keratin-type protein is the main constituent of the embryophore and that the hydrolysate of the embryophoric blocks was particularly positive for cystine. As the PFAS-reaction is not crucial enough, we tried also other methods but failed to obtain histochemical evidence of the presence of cystine and tryptophane. Interesting is the brilliant, red-violet staining with Ziehl-Neelsen's carbol-fuchsine, observed also by CAPRON and ROSE (1962) in the eggs of *Trh. saginatus*. The same staining reaction is given also by cestode hooks. The striking similarity in the properties of the substance of the hooks and the embryophore underlined by the same distinct argirophilia and osmophilia will be discussed in the chapter dealing with these structures. An acid fast staining in Ziehl - Neelsen's technique occurs also in the keratin of the hair cortex (MARGOLENA 1963) this being further evidence of the keratin-type protein in the embryophoric blocks. Confirmatory reactions for the presence of keratin in the embryophore of *Dipylidium caninum* were obtained by PENCE (1967). The ultrastructure of this species is different, as it does not originate from the embryophoric blocks but from two zones of numerous small embryophoric rods. The cement substance is of a different nature. Our findings do not confirm those by PAVLOVA (1965) that it consists of proteins and lipids. MEYMARIAN (1961)* concluded that the cement substance of the embryophore is nonproteinaceous in *E. granulosus*. The presence of glycogen in the inner layer of the embryophore on its external surface may also offer an explanation, because the original, granular layer in which the embryophoric blocks originate, contains much glycogen which disappears during the later development.

The analysis of the egg membrane confirms its high resistance to the external environment ensuring the relatively long survival of the oncosphere. The hatching of the embryo armed with 3 pairs of hooks involves two processes: the release of the hexacanth embryo from its membranes and the stimulation of the embryo to activity. In taeniid eggs, the capsule with the vitelline cell is very delicate and lost while still in the segment or in the faeces. In the intestinal tract of the intermediate host infected with these eggs, the hatching from the embryophore is affected by the digestion of the cement substance between the blocks. In a number of cestodes this occurs under the influence of pancreatin suggesting that this process is accomplished in the intestine. In an experiment with the eggs of *Trh. saginatus* SILVERMANN (1954a) found that the embryophore was not affected by pancreatin even after 30 hours, but could be disrupted in pepsin after 2—3 hours. This may indicate an adaptation of this species to the stomachs of ruminants. Other species can pass faster through the simple stomach of their intermediate hosts. It seems certain that intestinal factors together

---

*) Am. J. trop. Med. Hyg. 10 : 719—726, 1961.

with differences in the nature of the cement substance of the embryophore of various species are responsible for the fact that hatching and activating of the oncosphere can occur only in suitable intermediate hosts. Activation itself depends greatly on the presence of bile in the intestinal juice and also on its composition, because the bile factor is known to influence even the permeability of the oncospheral membrane. SILVERMAN (1954a) concluded that the oncospheral membrane in *Trh. saginatus* was lipoidal in nature. The activated oncosphere penetrates the intestinal wall with its embryonal hooks (their composition is described on p. 27) and with paired penetration glands, described by SILVERMAN (1954b) in *Trh. saginatus*. These glands are syncytial, giving a PAS-positive reaction which, however, is not destroyed by saliva. This indicates that the secretion is probably a mucopolysaccharide. The oncospheres penetrate the blood capillaries and are carried by the blood to their predilection sites. FROYD and ROUND (1960), on the other hand, found that cattle could be infected by subcutaneous or intramuscular injection of hatched oncospheres of *Trh. saginatus*. At the site of its final location, the oncosphere sheds its hooks mainly by expelling them from the body and changes into a mother bladder. From it, by progressive differentiation, does the cyclophyllidean larva — the cysticercus — develop. This will be described in the following chapter.

# Morphogenesis of the larval stage –
# the cysticercus

## 1. Transformation of the oncosphere into a mother bladder

Little information is available on the further development of the oncosphere after its location in the intermediate host. The embryo having shed its embryonal hooks represents an aggregation of cells. Mostly only its transformation into a bladder with a distinct doublelined membrane has been recorded. YOUNG (1908) making a detailed study of the very early stages of *C. pisiformis* concluded that this bladder consists of the loose syncytium of several parenchyma cells with a network of cytoplasmic processes and fibrils. The spaces within the cellular network seem to be filled with tissue fluid. In this developmental stage, the surface of the formation consists only of parenchyma. Later, the fibrils under the surface of the larva become arranged into two layers and gradually start to multiply and join into bundles. The cells start to concentrate more densely below this arrangement of the surface of the body to form the future subcuticular cell layer. Thin processes, running out of these cells, are in connection with the superficial fibrillar layer which, after being thickened by a further deposition of cement substance, differentiates on its surface a cuticular border of delicate hair-like processes. Some of the subcuticular cells differentiate into muscle cells and later form two layers of muscle fibrils lying perpendicular to each other. This differentiation of the bladder wall occurs simultanously with the formation of the central cavity of the mother bladder.

The embryo of *Hydatigera taeniaeformis* changes very quickly into a mother bladder. RAUM (1833, cit. BRAUN 1894 to 1900) found this transformation to occur on the 6th day or even earlier, KAN (1933, cit. ORIHARA 1962) observed this as soon as on the 3rd day. These bladders are covered with a thin wall and attain a diameter of less than 0·05 mm. It was not possible to trace histologically in these bladders the formation of the cavity. In agreement with these observations CRUSZ (1948b) found 10-day-old larvae as elongate or ovoid bladders measuring from 0·20—0·46 mm in diameter.

*C. cellulosae*, according to MOSLER (1864, cit. LEUCKART 1881—1887), after 8 days of infection appears as a bladder of more than 0·03 mm in diameter filled with a granular content. Larvae measuring 1 mm in diameter are already bladders filled with fluid, their differentiated wall measuring 7—10 µm. Leuckart described a 3-week-old *C. bovis* as a larva measuring 0·4—0·6 mm in length; the centre of the larva was filled with pale, non-nucleate pouches, which he considered to be transformed parenchyma cells. McIntosh and Miller (1960) depicted *C. bovis* up to the length of more than 1 mm as a bladder without a scolex-anlage. Silverman and Hulland (1961) noted in bladders of *C. bovis* measuring less than 0·5 mm a thin wall formed by a "multi-nucleated reticular tissue". Also Bott (1898) found *C. crassiceps* of 0·25 mm in diameter as distinct bladders, as did Anischenko (1953) who observed in *C. tenuicollis* a cavity in a bladder measuring less than 0·1 mm in diameter and also a wall composed of two to three layers of elongate, basophilic cells. On the other hand, quoting Leuckart, no true cavity can be found in such young larvae of this species. In all young stages of the cysticercus with an initial differentiation of the central cavity, the subcuticular layer of muscular fibrils crossing each other has already been developed and the shedding of the cuticle of the young larva may possibly follow after the differentiation of this layer.

In *C. pisiformis*, the central cavity is formed at a very late stage. Leuckart found a distinct differentiation of the wall in larvae measuring in length 0·5 mm and more. The bladder-wall is separated by a transformation of the parenchymatous cells (1·5 µm in diameter) into non-nucleated pouches measuring 6 µm, in the centre of the larva. However, the real cavity of the bladder is formed only in larvae measuring 4—5 mm in length by an accumulation of fluid in the centre of the larva. Potseluyeva (1953), in *C. pisiformis*, found this central cavity only in larvae which had attained a length of 7—10 mm.

We observed the differentiation of the wall of the mother bladder of *C. tenuicollis* measuring 2—3 mm in length and 0·5 mm in diameter. On the surface of the bladder we noted an already completely developed network of crossed muscle fibres. There was also a central cavity filled with a proteinic substance, coagulated by fixation into coarser granules. Also in the central cavity of some specimens we observed large, empty hollows measuring 15—40 µm in diameter lined with a distinct wall, while in other larvae the centre of their body consisted of a continuous network of septa. The hollows in this network were empty or filled with the remnants of a homogeneous proteinic substance. These findings represent the final stage in the development of the bladder cavity, originating from the liquifaction of the central portion of the parenchymatous larva, as this was recorded by Leuckart. As described, the wall of the mother bladder was formed by a 50 µm thick layer of still feebly differentiated cells.

In older larvae measuring 0·6—0·8 mm in diameter, the wall of the bladder is considerably thicker, measuring up to 150 µm and even more. The cellular elements are differentiated into a layer of elongate, subcuticular cells and into the principal layer of thin parenchyma, formed by a network of delicate fibres with very dispersed, spherical cells. In these larvae, the cells in the subcuticular layer are closely arranged and the surface layer, its nature being mostly that of neutral mucopolysaccharides, attains a thickness of 8 and even 9 µm. The features of the cuticle and subcuticula are the same as those of the zone of growth in the scolex of adult cysticerci, the surface of the cuticle being without fine, hairlike processes. In these larvae the ovoid formations of up to 50 μm in diameter, also present in the parenchyma of the wall, gave reactions of acid mucopolysaccharides. In view of the distinguishable nucleus, these seem to be cellular glands containing a secretion which might damage the parenchyma of the liver to clear the way for the passage of the cysticercus through this organ.

The young stages of *C. bovis*, measuring 0·8 and 1·3 mm, had a similarly differentiated bladder-wall and a cavity filled with a proteinic substance. The wall of the bladders of *C. crassiceps* measuring 1—2 mm in diameter represented the same final phase in the differentiation as the bladder-wall of the larvae with an entirely developed scolex and a secondarily diminished central cavity.

It clearly follows from these observations that the whole wall of the mother bladder resembles in its histological features the zone of growth, from which, in the later stage of the cysticercus, the scolex develops. The typical structure of the bladder-wall in older cysticerci with the paucity of subcuticular cells and the very delicate cuticle with fine, hairlike processes, is formed by the further differentiation of the mother bladder, apparently at the time of formation and further development of the scolex-anlage. The cuticle of the mother bladder resembles a secretion of the gland-like cells which, according to SCHILLER (1960) impregnates the fibrillar processes of the tapered, elongated, epithelially arranged subcuticular cells. The glandlike cells described by this author as being distributed throughout the bladder wall of unclearly identified cysticerci from the liver of *Tamiascirus hudsonicus*, could not be found by us in *C. tenuicollis*; we observed only the prominent glandular structures described in the foregoing text. The wall of the differentiated bladder of the cysti-cercus may, however, re-attain its primordial features in the case of its secondary proliferation as for example in the racemose form of *C. cellulosae*. Under these circumstances the histological structure of the bladder-wall is similar to the mother bladder, as this will be described later.

## 2.  Differentiation and development of the scolex-anlage

In the mother bladder with either a differentiated or still differentiating cavity, the latter applying to *C. pisiformis*, the scolex-anlage starts to develop only after the complete histological differentiation of the bladder-wall. In elongate, bi-polar larvae such as *C. crassiceps* and *C. pisiformis*, the germ centre becomes differentiated at one end, which we suggest calling the anterior end. In other cysticerci with a more spherical mother bladder, the original formation of the scolex-anlage is not so strictly confined to a certain site and the bi-polar shape of the larva is attained during the development of the scolex. In most cysticerci this process occurs in the third to fourth week of development. The size of the mother bladder varies without generally exceeding 1 mm in diameter.

Histologically, the origin of the scolex-anlage is characterized mainly by a proliferation of cells in the subcuticular layer. The accumulating cells form a local thickening of the bladder wall protruding into the central cavity (Fig. 2A). The basophilic cells having one or several nuclei, bear all the typical signs of cells in the active zone of growth, differing distinctly from the parenchymal cells which form the thin, fibrillar tissue under the layer of subcuticular cells. The cells on the surface of the whole growing scolex-anlage increase in number, draw closer and become arranged in parallel lines into a sheath of connective tissue character. This fibrous sheath separating the scolex from the cavity of the cysticercus, varies in appearance, make-up and thickness in the various species of cysticerci. In the literature this layer is known as the "receptaculum scolecis" although this term has been interpreted differently by the various writers. For Siebold the "receptaculum" represented the whole mother-bladder in which the scolex developed at a later stage. Moniez so designated the whole wall of the invaginated scolex-anlage in which the scolex differentiates. Also Leuckart in his description of *C. cellulosae* found that this layer, resembling connective tissue in its structure, separates directly the scolex of this cysticercus from the bladder-cavity.

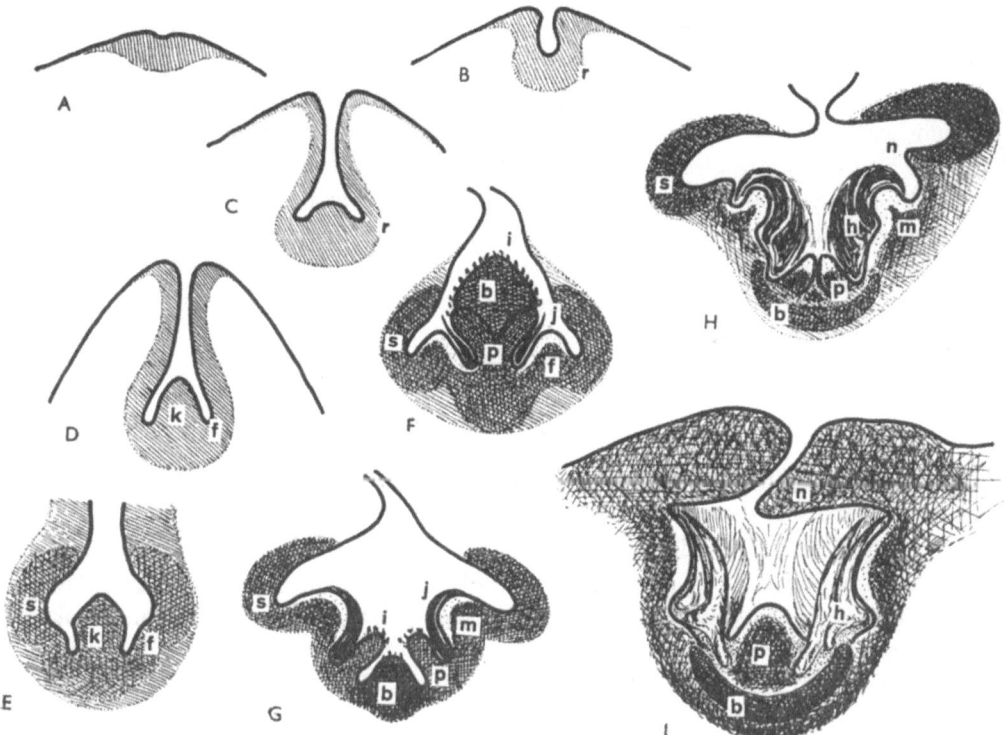

Fig. 2. Successive development of the invaginated scolex, the rostellum and hooks, schematized after Gläser and Crusz. k — rostellar cone; s — sucker; b — bulb; p — prebulbar region; f — circular furrow; i — hooklets; m — mountlike eminence with hypertrophic cuticle; j — primitive hook; r — receptaculum scolecis; h — definitive hooks; n — new elevation.

However, he also designated as "receptaculum" the continuation of this layer which runs into the folds of the bladder-wall, covers the scolex and forms a special vestibule (Vorhöhle). SCHAAF (1905) was in doubt about a special name for the separating connective tissue layer, which is so typical of the histological structure of every cysticercus. He proposed to reserve this term only for the description of the microscopic anatomy of *C. cellulosae*.

The surface cuticle invaginates very soon into the scolex-anlage (Fig. 2B). The scolex-cells are arranged into a thick subcuticular layer, consisting of several rows of densely packed cells. The invagination proceeds very quickly and results in the cavitation of the once solid cell-mass. The blind end of the hollow bud becomes enlarged forming thus a bottom, which is bordered by a circular furrow (Fig. 2C). The cell-proliferation is biggest under this floor of the hollow scolex-anlage and, consequently, the floor bulges upwards and the circular furrow deepens. Usually at the time when the scolex-anlage measures 1 mm in length, an elevation called the rostellar cone arises from this floor (Fig. 2D). Four shallow depressions occur laterally in the wall of the bud under which the cell-proliferation constitutes the anlage of the scolex-suckers (Fig. 2E).

In this way the rostellar cone develops in most cysticerci. A detailed description of this development in *C. crassiceps* was given by Gläser and his findings were confirmed by FREEMAN (1962). The first description of this development in *C. pisiformis* and in other cysticerci was given by Leuckart and his findings in *C. pisiformis* were confirmed by CRUSZ (1948b). An interesting deviation from these conditions was observed by Crusz in *Strobilocercus fasciolaris*. In BARTEL'S original description (1902) of the origin of the rostellar cone, the cone in this species as in other cysticerci starts to develop at the floor of the elongated invagination of the cuticle. Crusz, however, described this separation of the rostellar cone as occurring before the later elongation and sinking of the hollow bud into the mother bladder. His observation seems to be in agreement with GOLDSCHMIDT'S description (1900) of the development of the scolex-anlage in the echinococcus, although the scolices in this species differentiate under other circumstances than those in the cysticerci.

In a later developmental stage, the rostellar cone becomes greatly enlarged especially in its mid-portion. The circular furrow between the cone and the differentiating suckers deepens and reduces the base of the cone, which connects it with the floor of the hollow bud. At the same time, the cuticle grows and forms an invagination on its wide, lateral circumference which, even on the surface of the rostellar cone, indicates its internal division into a double cone. The upper proliferation centre in the pointed portion is called the bulb, the lower centre in its narrowed base is called the prebulbar region (Fig. 2F).

By the subsequent extensive growth of the prebulbar region the bulb sinks gradually into the underlying mass of cells and comes to lie on the floor of the scolex-anlage (Fig. 2G). There it flattens into a dish-shaped formation, which is the anlage of the rostellar sucker. The hypertrophical prebulbar region, having closed over the bulb, now forms the rostellar peak surrounded by the enlarged lateral area. This developed from the original circular furrow separating the rostellar cone on the floor of the bud (Fig. 2H). This area is separated from the remaining surface of the cavity of the scolex-anlage by the scolex suckers. In a later stage of rostellar development the hooks of the cysticercus appear in the cuticular substance, formed abundantly in this area.

## 3.  Hooks, their origin, shape and composition

At the time of further differentiation and transformation of the rostellar cone, the thickened cuticle covering most of the bulb and prebulbar region bears minute filiform and conical hooklets, which are present also in the furrow around the cone up to the suckers developing from the shallow depressions (Fig. 2F). These hooklets are formed by the cementing of groups of superficial cuticular hairs, which Young considered as being the continuation of fibrils of subcuticular and parenchymal cells. At the time when the prebulbar region closes over the bulb, these minute spines disappear. Only in the deepening furrow between the prebulbar region and on the new, high, mount-like eminence of subcuticular cells, which displaced the sucker-anlagen, do these hooklets attain a considerably larger size. Being situated in the furrow they take on a sickle-shaped appearance, bending hook-like in conformity with the width and depth of the fold (Fig. 2G). These hollow claw-like formations are the anlage around which the blade of the definitive hook will be formed. The curved inner edge of the primitive hook lies directly on the mount-like eminence. The hypertrophy of the cuticle in the wall of the eminence adjoining the hooks is very striking; the primitive hooks now practically completely covered by it are fixed by their lower ends to the bottom of the bordering furrow. This widens and its cuticle becomes noticeably hypertrophic (Fig. 2H). A newly formed elevation at the edge of the suckers practically closes the cavity above the coalesced prebulbar mount (Fig. 2I). This space is filled with a hypertrophic cuticle in which the hooks attain their definitive shape by the deposition of a specific substance on the outside of the primordial primitive hooks. Their base originates in the widened furrow beyond the prebulbar region and the dimension and shape of this furrow and of the cuticular elevations evidently influence the shape and the size of the hooks in the various cysticercus species. GLÄSER (1909) mentioned an unusual hypertrophy of the cuticle, which was permeated by vacuoles of different staining properties; these were also described by CRUSZ (1947, 1948b). The specific nature of this cuticle is closely related to its function in hook-formation.

The completely developed hook consists of a blade with a medulla and a cortex layer and of a base. The base of the hook composed of an anterior extension (handle) and a posterior extension (guard) is uneven, homogeneous and sunk into the cuticular layer. In staining histological sections of the hook, the complicated structure of the base is defined. The homogeneous central portion is of the same nature as the cortex layer of the blade, while the surface of the base is covered with a layer of a different nature.

When examining the hook by phase contrast and with various histological methods, its medulla looked mostly like a cavity, appearing sometimes as if containing also a fibrous structure stainable with eosin. Its delimitation from the cortex layer was most uneven. With PAS and Best's carmine either its delimitation line or the entire medullar part became pale coloured. Also CRUSZ (1948b) described the differentiation of the inner "membrane" by various methods.

The substance forming the cortex layer of the blade and a major portion of the base is very distinct in its nature. It is refractory to staining with a number of histological methods and has its own greenish colour which depends on its high refractive index. However, it stains yellow with picric acid by van Gieson's method, yellowish-green with Hale's method and feebly red by Goldner. Characteristic is the blue to bluish-green colour in the regressive staining after Giemsa, in which it is possible to demonstrate selectively the hooks of the cestodes, as described in a previous paper (ŠLAIS 1960). Of importance also is the fact that the hooks always stain various shades of brown with methods for the reduction of silver nitrate (e.g. after Kossa, Gomori, Masson). Histochemical reactions of the cortex layer were found to be brilliant blue with the PFA-AB method; however, an indistinct staining was obtained in the tests for the detection of SH-groups. In a procedure after Ziehl-Neelsen the hooks colour an intense purple. From the foregoing account it is possible to conclude that the main portion of cestode hooks, i.e. the cortex layer of the blade and most of the base are formed by a scleroprotein, which is very resistant to the effect of reagents, is highly refractive and contains an abundance of SS-groups. Reactions for tyrosin, tryptophane and arginine were negative.

The layer on the surface of the hook base is of a different chemical composition. With various methods it stains only as a substance of basophilic character. It is interesting to note that this layer is thickest at the transition of the base into the blade, there forming a distinctly separated sheath into which the blade is inserted. Towards the bottom of the base this sheath reduces until it fuses with it. With Giemsa's method it stains an intense blue, turning violet at the upper edge. An intense, positive colouring is obtained in Millon's reaction and in the detection of SH-groups, a slightly positive colouring in Sakaguchi's reaction. With Goldner's method it colours bright red, with Hale's method green. All these findings indicate that the protein in the surface of the hook-base is of a different composition mainly in that it contains tyrosin (but not tryptophane), cystein and arginine. This layer seems to be of a more complicated nature; the PAS-positivity, the green colouring with Hale's method and metachromasia with Giemsa suggest also the presence of a mucopolysaccharide. This layer communicates closely with the proper connective tissue sheath of the hook, formed by a parenchyma which colours red with van Gieson, green with Goldner and in which Gomori's method demonstrates a network of argyrophilic fibres.

The onset of hook development was discovered in young stages of *C. crassiceps*. The cuticle of the prebulbar region of the scolex-anlage was covered with numerous minute hooklets and later with considerably larger, proper hooks. However, these hooks having neither an increased refractive index nor being of the typical shape, appeared like elongate, pointed cones, which were strikingly eosinophilic. In *Sc.* (= *Strobilocercus*) *fasciolaris* of a more advanced stage of development we discovered the start of sclerotization of these primitive hooks. The original hook substance although still distinctly eosinophilic, was clearly interspersed with vacuoles and its surface appeared to be impregnated. The eosinophilic part stained also as an acid mucopolysaccharide with the combined Hale-PAS method and metachromatically with Giemsa's stain. The surface layer, however, when stained with Giemsa, became the typical blue of the fully developed hook, its refractive index and the histological staining reactions being also identical with those of the hook. Our finding supports Gläser's conclusion that the definitive hook is formed by the apposition of a highly refractive substance to the surface of the small, conical elevations of the cuticle and not by a deposition on the inner surface of these hooklets as suggested by LEUKKART (1879—1886). During sclerotization of the hook the original anlage degenerates and the medulla originating from it may retain some particles of the original substance. These remnants may be responsible for the positive reaction to polysaccharides in completely developed hooks, in which the medulla disappears as also observed by LOGACHEV (1959) in *C. cellulosae*. Degenerated cell elements are certainly not present in the disappearing medulla as held by this writer and fibrillar structures which form the original cuticular points by cementing are more likely to be detected in them. This was confirmed by YOUNG (1908).

Our findings and those of other investigators show that the hooks of cestodes are highly differentiated organs, which finish their morphogenesis as early as in the cysticercus stage. They are formed by a scleroprotein containing a high amount of sulphur. The histological comparison of this scleroprotein with the cortex layer of vertebrate hairs revealed a considerable similarity, which was confirmed by their equal reaction to Ziehl-Neelsen's stain. MARGOLENA (1963) drew attention to the high affinity for stain of the hair cortex in contrast to the unstained medulla. Also the chemical and optical properties of both substances were found to be the same. The specific chemical structure of cestode hooks is responsible for the selective blue staining with Giemsa; the keratin of the hair cortex stains the same blue. Therefore, it is not surprising to find also similarities in the histogenesis of both structures: the medulla of the fully developed hair is hollow and contains remnants of degenerate cells; the medulla of the hook is also hollow at a later stage and contains remnants of fibrillary structures. A histochemical character of the hair sheath is the presence of tyrosin (but not tryptophane), arginine and SH-groups, which applies also to the sheath at the base of the hook showing that the processes occurring during the development of the keratin of the cortex and of the scleroproteid of the hooks are alike. Their great similarity is further confirmed by the high contents of unbonded or weakly bonded reducing agents which affect silver nitrate and cause a brown colouring of the hooks and of the hair cortex. These substances may be polyphenols as suggested by MONNÉ (1960) who considered their participation in the formation of exoplasmatic structures in invertebrates and vertebrates to be of great importance. In his opinion they are nonspecific inhibitors of enzymes and he believed them to be bonded in glucosides or esters of acid mucopolysaccharides. In a complex with protein they are responsible for the high resistance of the cuticles and even of the egg-covers of some nematodes. According to our findings (ŠLAIS 1964) their substance is related to that of cestode hooks.

One point, however, needs clarification and that is the presence of polysaccharides in the main substance of cestode hooks, until recently considered to be a chitin. DOLLFUS (1942) was the first to draw attention to the staining of tetrarhynchid hooks, which was not indicative of a chitin. CRUSZ (1947) in his microchemical studies of the hook substance in *Sc. fasciolaris* obtained a negative reaction for chitin and concluded on the basis of positive results from various other tests (Biuret, Millon, Sakaguchi, the xanthoproteinic reaction and the method with lead acetate) that this substance is strongly suggestive of a scleroprotein with high sulphur contents. Later CRUSZ (1948b) performed various well-known tests, also using histological sections of the hooks of other cysticerci and thus demonstrated a difference between the blade and the base of the hook. In these tests even he obtained positive results with Schulze's reaction for chitin in the blade. The hooks were entirely resistant to peptic and tryptic digestion. He found a birefringence in the blade, but not in the base of the hook. The positive test for proteins was considerably greater in the base, but Crusz failed to note that only the thin layer covering the base is different in its composition and not the whole base substance. It will be necessary to reconfirm the finding of a positive reaction for chitin in the blade. GALLAGHER (1964) analyzing biochemically with paper chromatography a sufficient number of hooks of the echinococcus did not detect glucosamine or sugar. In view of the composition of the amino-acids he concluded that the hook substance is a keratin-type protein slightly different from the typical keratin of vertebrates.

The hooks of the oncosphere are as complicated in structure as those of the cysticercus. The part within the body of the oncosphere extending from base to collar, is covered by a connective tissue sheath with muscles attached to it. COLLIN (1968) called the special superficial layer, found by electron microscopy, the outer granular layer. There is no information available as yet on its chemical composition. The main middle fibrous layer of high electron density extends from the base to the hook tip. Collin maintains that its fibrils are of similar size to those occurring in keratin. Also PENCE (1967) found the same positive reaction for keratin in the hooks of the oncosphere of *Dipylidium caninum* although it was slightly less intense. However, we were able to show that in the eggs of *Trh. saginatus* the hooks of the oncosphere stained very strongly with PAA-AF. Nothing is known about the composition of the inner core, which appears by electron microscopy as a laminated crystalline-like material. To study the histochemistry of the oncospheral hooks during embryogenesis seems, therefore, of great importance although the minute size of these hooks will make this study most difficult.

# Morphology of *Cysticercus cellulosae* and *Cysticercus bovis*

## 1. Introduction

A typical character of the fully developed cysticercus is the differentiation of its body into the bladder and the parenchymatous portion. In the various species the bladder differs in size and shape. There is also a difference between the histological structure of the bladder wall and that of the parenchymatous portion with the invaginated scolex. The suckers and the moderately elevated rostellum with the hooks are placed at the blind termination of the spiral canal inside the parenchymatous portion. The parenchyma being thickest around the invaginated scolex, is made up of relatively horizontally arranged fibrils and of distinct, minute, spindle-shaped cells. The layer covering this portion plays an important part during the evagination of the scolex and contains a system of muscle fibrils. The folded wall of the invaginated canal is covered with a high, relatively homogeneous cuticle with numerous marked grooves. More parenchyma with typical calcareous corpuscles is present in the folds of the wall. In cysticerci localized in the musculature, the parenchymatous portion of the larva is completely closed in by the bladder cavity. The surface of the parenchymatous portion facing the bladder cavity is lined only with a fibrous tissue (receptaculum) with elongate cells arranged in parallel. At the opening of the spiral canal on to the bladder surface, its wall changes its histological appearance when coalescing with the bladder wall.

The fully developed bladders of *C. cellulosae* and *C. bovis*, at this stage capable of infecting man, are very much alike both being ovoid to pointed in shape. Inside the translucent bladder wall, mostly midway, lies close to the surface of the wall a massive, opaque, spherical formation representing the invaginated scolex. There is little difficulty in distinguishing a developed *C. cellulosae* from a *C. bovis*, because the scolex of the former is armed with hooks of a typical shape, their number being 22—32, usually 26—28 while there are no hooks on the scolex of *C. bovis*. Also the morphological structure of *C. cellulosae* is different from that of *C. bovis*. In *C. cellulosae* (Fig. 3) the surface of the bladder-wall does not pass through the opening in its wall directly into the spiral canal leading to the suckers and rostellum, as it does in *C. bovis*, but the wall turns at the edge of the opening, enveloping most of the parenchymatous portion without significantly changing its thickness. When it has almost reached the deepest part of the invaginated portion it becomes confluent with the parenchyma. The bottom of the resulting slit is slightly folded and covers

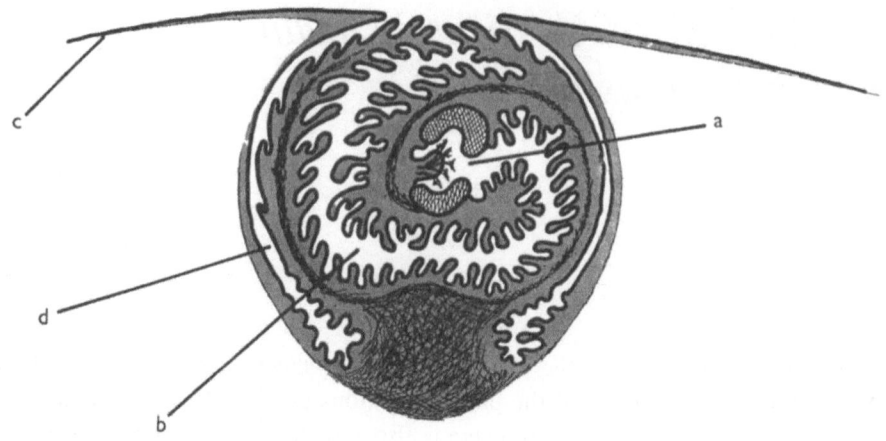

Fig. 3. Schematic illustration of the structure of the invaginated portion of *C. cellulosae*. a — invaginated scolex; b — spiral canal; c — bladder wall; d — vestibule.

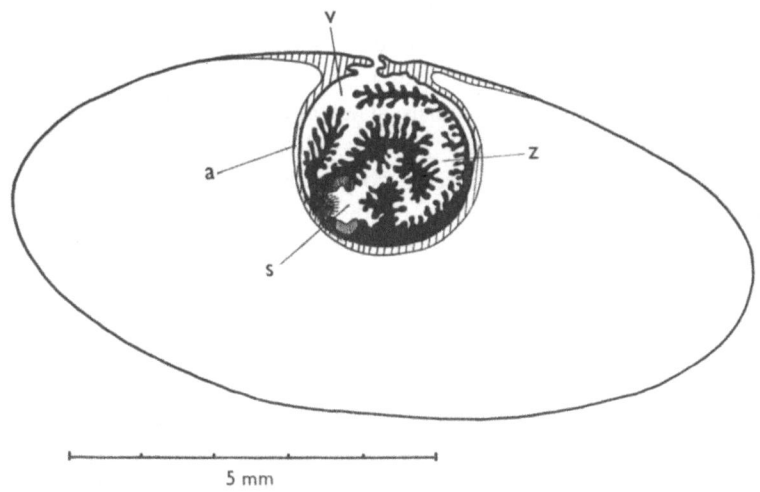

Fig. 4. Schematic survey of *C. cellulosae* after Leuckart. s — invaginated scolex; z — spiral canal; v — space of vestibule; a — wall of vestibule.

a knob-like area in which the parenchymatous tissue of the cysticercus is thickest. In these places the cuticle lining the slit-like space between the parenchymatous portion and the outermost cover, which is actually a continuation of the bladder-wall, passes on to the surface of the parenchymatous portion. LEUCKART (1879—1886) used the term "Vorhöhle" to designate this slit-like space (Fig. 4). Into it opens the spiral canal (Leuckart and other writers call it "Zwischenstück") leading to the invaginated scolex. On the outer pole of the invaginated portion visible through the opening in the bladder-wall, the cuticle now passes into the folds of the spiral canal

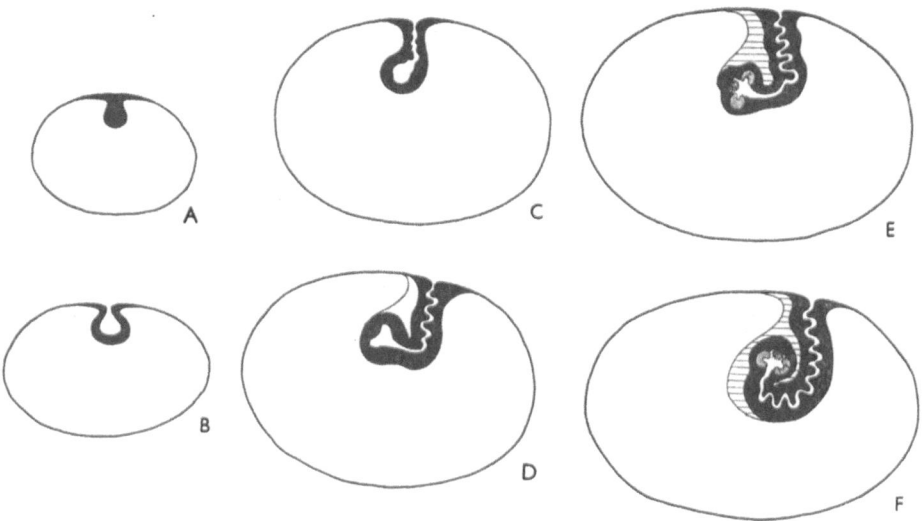

Fig. 5. Scheme of the development of *C. cellulosae* after Leuckart.

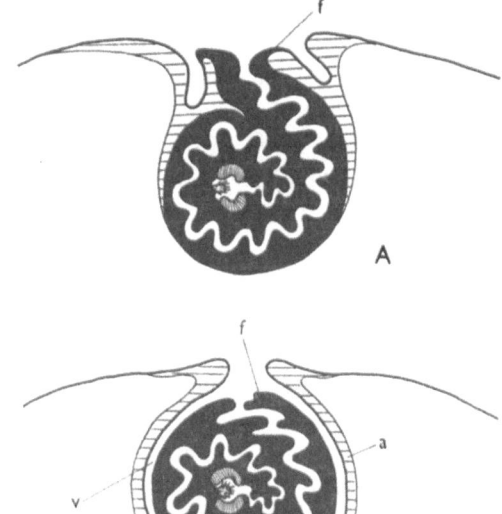

Fig. 6. Formation of the vestibule in *C. cellulosae* according to Leuckart. A — initial folding of the bladder wall at the opening of the spiral canal; B — fully developed vestibule; f — opening of the spiral canal; v — space of the vestibule; a — wall of the vestibule.

leading to the suckers and the rostellum with the hooks. This shows that the spiral canal in *C. cellulosae* is not communicating directly with the surface of the bladder.

LEUCKART (1879—1886) in his generally accepted view on the development of *C. cellulosae* maintained that the mother bladder originates first; then follows the differentiation of the scolex and the parallel growth of both portions (Fig. 5). Leuckart at first found no explanation for the origin of the vestibule (Vorhöhle), suggesting later that it may be a mere fold originating around the primary opening of the spiral canal onto the bladder-surface and deepening steadily so that it actually separates the entire invaginated portion (Fig. 6). He considers it, however, to be an integral part of this opening, which only later becomes deeply folded. While studying its histological structure we found this outer covering to be similar to the bladder wall, having almost nothing in common with the invaginated portion and, moreover, the cuticle lining the vestibule, to form the transition from the cuticle of the bladder-surface to that of the spiral canal. The results of our studies of young stages of cysticerci suggest another explanation for the origin of the vestibule, which may contribute to the knowledge of the development of *C. cellulosae* and *C. bovis*.

## 2. Morphogenesis of *Cysticercus cellulosae*

The four youngest stages of cysticerci from a human brain were oval formations of about 3 mm in diameter. The moderately spiral canal leading to the already completely developed scolex with the suckers, rostellum and hooks, opened in folds into one end of the formation. The hooks typical of *C. cellulosae* numbered 26 (13 bigger and 13 smaller hooks). The surface of the spiral canal was folded. The formation was covered with a smooth, distinct cuticle, the parenchyma contained numerous calcareous corpuscles and trunks of fibrous and muscle tissue characteristic of the invaginated portion of the completely developed cysticercus. On the end lying opposite to the opening of the spiral canal the parenchymatous portion of the formation was attenuated into a neck covered with a deeply folded cuticle and then passed into the bladder. The parenchyma of the neck consisted of fibrous tissue with few calcareous corpuscles, but without well-defined ducts. The parenchymatous portion including the neck measured 2 mm. The thicker wall of the bladder was histologically typical in structure. It did not contain calcareous corpuscles and its surface was covered with wart-like protrusions, appearing as undulations in section. The histological differentiation of both portions was the same as that of the completely developed cysticerci. The bladders of these four cysticerci were different in size and shape. In one case the bladder occupied only a hole in the brain tissue and was lying close to the parenchymatous portion (Fig. 7). In another only the neck was sunk into the bladder cavity, the rest of the parenchymatous portion was still uncovered by the bladder. In the third case the bladder was dish-shaped and the parenchymatous portion was slightly recessed into it, leaving one side completely uncovered. In the fourth parasite the parenchymatous portion was covered up to one half of its length by the bladder (Plate I, Fig. 1).

In another observation we found 8 cysticerci, in which the bladder had changed from an appendage of the parenchymatous portion with the invaginated scolex into a coat-like envelope, leaving uncovered only the small portion with the opening of the spiral canal. The diameter (3 mm) of these stages was the same as that of the four previously described cysticerci. In some of the forms only the small aperture round the opening of the spiral canal remained uncovered by the enveloping bladder (Plate I, Fig. 2). In these we found a developed covering of the parenchymatous portion, a vestibule and its opening onto the bladder surface. The volume of the blad-

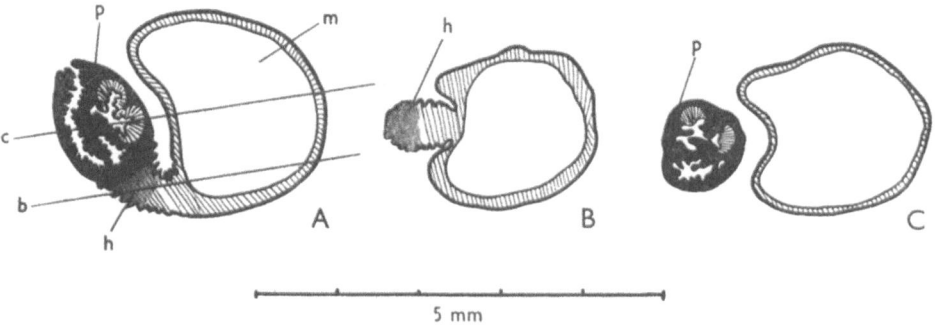

Fig. 7 Schematic illustration of the young stage of *C. cellulosae* from the brain of man. A — reconstruction of a longitudinal section showing the fully differentiated parenchymatous portion and the still separated bladder of the cysticercus; B and C — sections through the same cysticercus on a horizontal level; c — plane of section C; d — plane of section B; p — parenchymatous portion; h — neck; m — bladder.

der was relatively small and its shape irregular. The slightly spherical parenchymatous portion of these forms measured up to 2 mm in diameter. The diameter of the whole cysticercus was 3—4 mm. The wall of the vestibule, i.e. the proper covering of the parenchymatous portion, was very thin. The cuticle lining its inner surface was of the same type as that along the edge of the enveloping folds of the bladder. At the point of transition of the two surfaces we found solitary calcareous corpuscles in the parenchyma, which occupied most parts of the still solid folds of the bladder.

Most of the parasites from the circular cavities in the brain were spherical in shape, measuring mostly 5 mm in diameter. In most of them the outermost covering of the parenchymatous portion was developed. The only signs differentiating them from the typical *C. cellulosae* in the musculature were the smaller size of their bladder and their spherical shape, while the size of the parenchymatous portion of their body was that of a fully developed cysticercus, i.e. more than 3 mm in diameter. In 20 parasites this portion, but not the bladder, was found to be at a different stage of calcification.

The morphology of the described forms indicates that the bladder starts to overgrow the parenchymatous portion of the body with the invaginated scolex only after this portion has completed its development. In this way the typical *C. cellulosae* is formed. This developmental process was confirmed in two parasites located under the ependyma. The growing parasite bulged into the chamber; later its capsule under the ependyma became very thin, started to become necrotic and finally ruptured. The portion with the invaginated scolex protruded through the cleft and continued in its growth without changing its original appearance. The bladder having got stuck in the subependymal hole and lost its relationship with the parenchymatous portion of the body, also continued in its growth, thereby forming various folds and lobes (Fig. 8). A similar development was observed in one of the three parasites, which

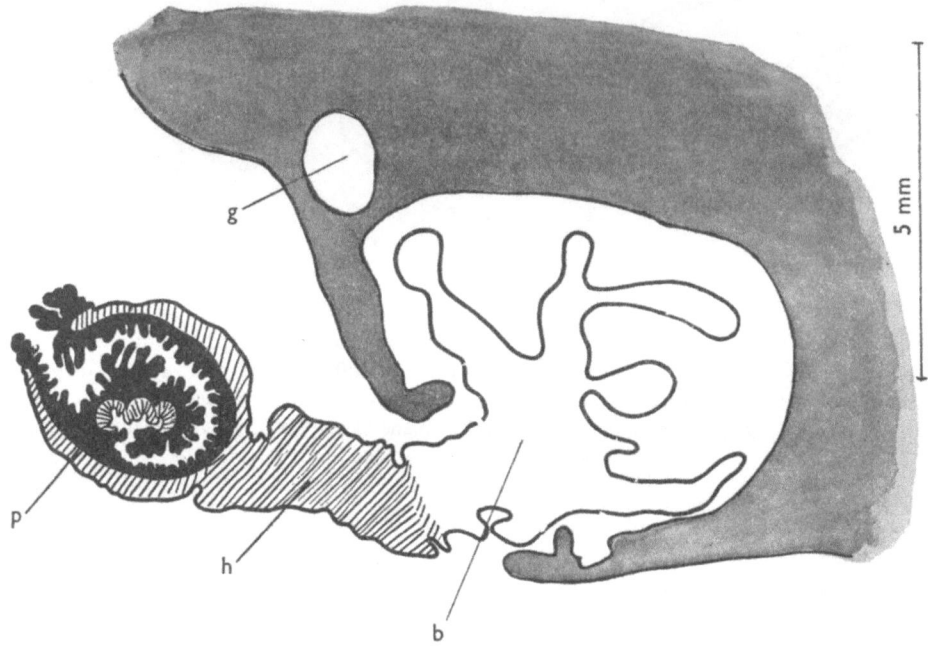

Fig. 8. Schematic illustration of a cysticercus in subependymal localization trapped in the ruptured wall of a cavity. The bladder and the parenchymatous portion developed independently. p — parenchymatous portion; h — neck; b — bladder; g — vessel.

were lying in closely adjoining holes. Also here the necrotic capsule had broken apart and the protruded parenchymatous portion of the cysticercus was found wedged between the two other bladders.

Our finding shows that the overgrowing of the parenchymatous portion of the body by the proliferating bladder can occur only in a closed-in space, which is a primary condition for the origin of a natural relationship between the invaginated portion and the bladder.

While studying a massive brain cysticercosis we also observed 4 larvae without an outermost covering and therefore, the whole surface of the parenchymatous portion was in direct contact with the fluid in the cavity of the bladder. The spiral canal differing in no way from that of other cysticerci, passed from the scolex directly to the bladder-surface. The morphology of these larvae was found to be in agreement with the view of Leuckart. The spiral canal did not form such a concentrated spherical formation as in a typical *C. cellulosae*, but was much more spread out. Histologically the actual opening of this canal was formed by a short part without calcareous corpuscles and its wall was found to be of the same structure as that of the bladder, which is similar to the situation in older forms of *C. bovis*. These bladders measured 3·5—5 mm in diameter. Their invaginated portion was 1·5 mm long.

Also in cysticerci from the musculature of swine, the number of hooks which are typical for *C. cellulosae*, was 13 + 13 = 26. The bladders were mostly ovoid to elongate, often of considerable volume. The vestibule and the outermost covering of the parenchymatous portion was developed in all larvae (Plate XII, Fig.1). The spiral canal, however, was mostly longer than that of the cysticerci from the brain cysticercosis. The folds in the wall of this canal were more elaborate and thus the structure of the parenchymatous portion was more complicated. The largest bladders were 12 mm long and 4 mm wide, the diameter of the invaginated portion was 2—3 mm. In some of the cysticerci the bladder had not yet completely overgrown the parenchymatous portion. Its shape was irregular and especially its proliferating parts were often still solid (Plate XIII, Fig. 1, Plate XXII, Fig. 1). In histological sections of the musculature it was possible to demonstrate that the bladder may attain an elongate shape by growing sideways into the lymphatic capillaries which are capable of considerable dilation.

From our finding it is evident that in *C. cellulosae* the invaginated scolex and the spiral canal originate in the parenchymatous portion of the elongated larval body. The growing bladder gradually overgrows the parenchymatous portion and the typical cysticercus is formed. MONIEZ (1880) in his description of *C. cellulosae* depicted this process of overgrowing of the portion with the invaginated scolex, which measured even more than 3 mm in length. In our material from a brain cysticercosis, such large formations were always completely covered by the bladder. The size given by Moniez for the parenchymatous portion and his observation of the solid structure of the proliferating part of the bladder are closer to some of our own findings in a muscle cysticercosis of swine. However, he figured and described this developmental stage as an isolated observation not preceded by any other developmental forms, because his material must have been incomplete as is evident also from his description of other cysticerci. Therefore, his accurate observation was not accepted by Leuckart, and SCHAAF (1906) declared it to be speculative and most improbable. Although LEUCKART (1863) mentioned in his study of smaller stages of *C. cellulosae* a bladder 0·8 mm long, he described the larvae as being attenuated towards the scolex anlage with a thickened surface from which the actual anlage protruded in wart-like fashion. Hence it follows that these were elongate larvae, but of a smaller size. Also his evidence suggests that he was dealing with incomplete and extremely variable material although it was greater in quantity than that of Moniez. Also OSTERTAG (1895) described in a 60-day-old *C. cellulosae* with developed hooks and suckers a scolex-anlage which was the size of a pea and was raised above the bladder surface.

While studying a cysticercus in swine, Böhm (1917) found in addition to normally developed bladders with the invaginated portion many with an unusual feature. These bladders were located in the connective tissue between the muscle fibres of the myocard at the base of the tendons and the papillary muscles of medium and smaller size. The invaginated scolex with the spiral canal was found at one end of the bladder which was heart-shaped and connected with the scolex portion by an attenuated neck. Böhm termed this form the "Flammenherzform der Schweinefinne". In this form the bladder had evidently not overgrown the otherwise completely developed invaginated portion. Christiansen (1932) observed cysticerci in cysts from the musculature of deer, which were very similar to C. cellulosae except that the invaginated scolex in some smaller larvae was located at one pole and that the bladder was distinctly smaller. This evidence from the literature and our findings suggest that in C. cellulosae a state persists in which the parenchymatous portion with the scolex passes only into the bladder without being closed-in by it. Generally, this state represents only a certain developmental stage of the cysticercus. The development of the cysticercus is not uniform and Leuckart himself observed a slower growth of cysticerci from the brain than of cysticerci from the musculature, generally finding in one organ bladders of various size and at different developmental stages. Most remarkable seems, therefore, his observation of a scolex-anlage with the differentiated organs measuring 1·3 by 1·3 mm while the bladder was more than 6 mm long. However, our observations suggest that irregularities in the development of the cysticercus may sometimes be caused by an excessive growth and differentiation of the scolex as compared with that of the bladder. Such fast development of the scolex can be noted in a massive infestation wherein the equally fast progress of tissue reaction of the intermediate host is responsible for a relatively sudden dystrophic calcification of the scolex, but not of the bladder. The decisive factor influencing the morphology of C. cellulosae is the site in which the parasite develops. Jakobson (1907) found in a massive cysticercosis not only parasites similar to those in our observations, but also an entrance canal originating from the commencing growth and enlargement of the bladder. Also the cavities and the capsules are consistent with our findings. However, his belief that the capsules are, in fact, the original wall of blood vessels in which their three components are still distinguishable, was firmly rejected some time ago. Also the photomicrographs Silverman and Hulland (1961) added to their study on the morphology of C. cellulosae from the musculature of swine and of C. bovis from the musculature of sheep give evidence of the secondary development of the bladder. The same conclusions can be drawn from the photomicrograph of C. cellulosae in a cysticercosis of man in the textbook by Craig and Faust (1951).

# 3.  Morphogenesis of *Cysticercus bovis*

In all our observations *C. bovis* appeared as an ovoid bladder measuring mostly 9—10 mm in length and 5 mm in width. The surface of the bladder of cysticerci isolated from the musculature showed characteristic protuberances. In young cysticerci the wall was translucent, in older cysticerci of a brown colour. The invaginat-

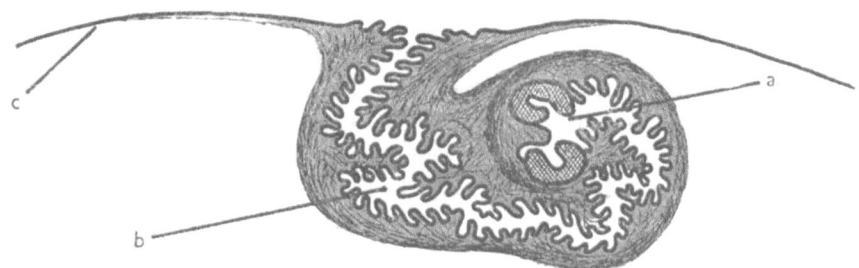

Fig. 9. Schematic illustration of the structure of the invaginated portion of *C. bovis*. a — invaginated scolex; b — spiral canal; c — bladder wall.

ed portion opened into the middle of the elongate bladder and in only one instance did we find it to open at one pole of the bladder. Its size was variable (larger in older cysticerci up to 3 mm in diameter) pear-shaped, the wider base facing the bladder cavity (Fig. 9). The spiral canal was less complicated than that of *C. cellulosae*; its wall was less folded. The pear-shaped invaginated portion in older cysticerci originates from an elongation of the spiral canal at the site, where it opens onto the bladder surface through the continued growth of the wall. In this way a new part opening onto the surface and called entrance canal is formed, which differs histologically from the spiral canal (Plate II, Fig. 3). Its excessive development changes the usual morphology of the cysticercus and prevents the evagination of the scolex. The parenchyma of the invaginated portion in *C. bovis* is closely packed with calcareous corpuscles (Plate XXI, Fig. 3) and contains little fibrous tissue. Hence it follows that this is actually only the parenchyma of the wall of the spiral canal and not the parenchymatous formation with the spiral canal as in *C. cellulosae*. In its histological structure the wall of the entrance canal is in keeping with that of the bladder wall and does not contain any calcareous corpuscles (Plate XXI, Fig. 4).

We found repeatedly cysticerci in which the opening of the spiral canal was prominently elevated above the level of the bladder wall, whereby the whole elevated portion was covered with the same cuticle as that in the canal (Plate II, Fig. 1). Sometimes, the distal end of the invaginated portion with the suckers covered with a more distinct layer of connective fibre, was connected with the bladder wall by a thin parenchyma. Twice we discovered anomalous forms, in which the invaginated portion was not sunk completely into the bladder. One of its sides was covered with the same cuticle as that on the surface of the spiral canal, the bladder wall forming there a kind of vestibule (Plate II, Fig. 2). However, this proved to be only a passive recession of one side of the invaginated portion into the bladder cavity caused by the pressure of the fibrous encapsulation and not by an active proliferation of the bladder as in *C. cellulosae*. Once we found an old *C. bovis* in which the parenchymatous portion was permanently connected with the bladder by a short constricted portion.

We never discovered young larvae of *C. bovis* at the earliest stage of scolex development. Moniez (1880), however, described even this cysticercus as being 3 mm long elongate, in which the anterior portion represents the developed, invaginated scolex and the posterior portion the developing bladder. The finding of a spindle-shaped larva was recorded by Leuckart (1880) in a cysticercus of 0·8 mm in length, by Silverman and Hulland (1961) in a cysticercus measuring 0·8 mm in length and 0·3 mm in width and by Ostertag (1897) in a cysticercus of 4 mm in length and 2 mm in width. In the descriptions of these authors, the cysticercus is a bladder with a relatively thin wall and with a scolex-anlage developing inside the bladder as a small elevation in its wall. This is in accord with the description by Hertwig (1891) and a more recent observation by McIntosh and Miller (1960), while Leuckart stated he had found this anlage in a still solid parenchymatous larva. Conflicting data are also recorded by various writers who have described the size of the fully developed invaginated scolex. McIntosh and Miller still depicted the invaginated portion as a solid mass bulging out prominently from the bladder even in a larva measuring 3 × 2·5 mm, while Dewhirst et al. (1963) considered similar forms to be the starting phase of scolex evagination.

## 4. Morphogenesis of the other cysticerci

Some information on the development of other cysticerci in which the parenchymatous portion is not lying inside the bladder cavity, might contribute to a better understanding of the complicated conditions in the development of *C. cellulosae* and *C. bovis* (Fig. 10). Dithyridium — our specimens were obtained from the subcutaneous region of a muskrat — is a parenchymatous larva with a typical invaginated scolex and a spiral canal without a cavity inside its body, but only an indication of a vacuolation of cells at one of its poles, which is very similar to the changes occurring in the cells of the central part of the mother bladder of other cysticerci during the onset of differentiation of its cavity. Particularly variable is *C. crassiceps*, which we discovered repeatedly in the abdominal cavity of *Microtus arvalis* in the most varying shapes and sizes. At the earliest stage it develops from a thin bladder with a scolex differentiating at one of the poles. Later, as the cysticerci grow older, the spiral canal distends and suppresses the bladder cavity. Braun (1894—1900) actually mentioned the possibility of finding all kinds of forms from mere bladders to fully developed cysticerci, in which almost the whole cavity is occupied by the developing scolex anlage. *C. pisiformis* retains its elongate larval shape up to a length of 4—5 mm, at which time the differentiation of the suckers and the rostellum has almost been completed; the development of the bladder at its posterior portion starts at a later stage. Also *C. tenuicollis* grows very quickly into the shape of an elongate bladder, its anterior portion soon becoming occupied by the developing scolex. In some intermediate hosts the bladder of this species may by far outgrow

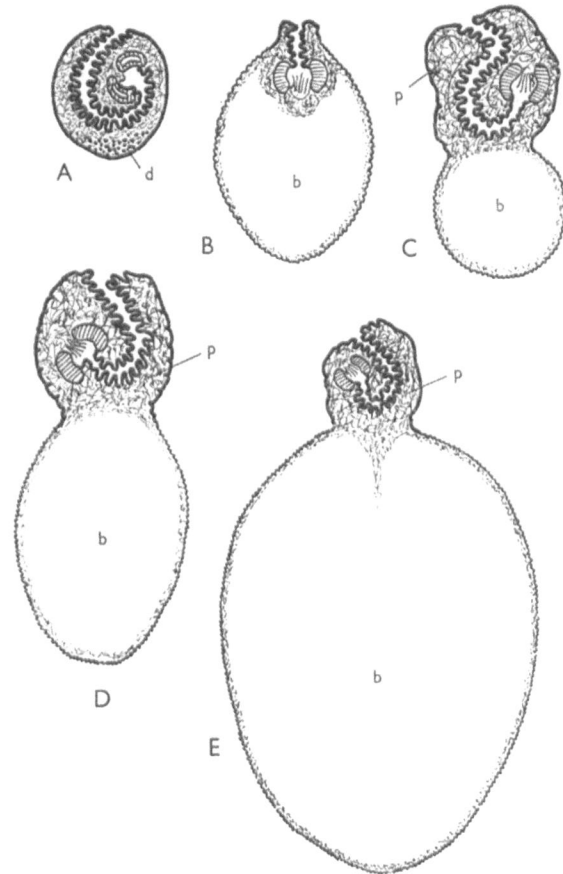

Fig. 10. Schematic illustration of the structure of other cysticerci. A — dithyridium, parenchymatous larva without a bladder; B — young *C. crassiceps* with a not yet developed invaginated portion. C — *C. crassiceps* with a fully developed parenchymatous portion occupying the former cavity of the bladder; D — *C. pisiformis*; E — *C. tenuicollis*; d — differentiation of the vacuoles at one pole of the larval body; p — parenchymatous portion; b — bladder.

the size of the parenchymatous portion with the invaginated scolex. In this connection it is interesting to note that all these types of cysticerci with or without a bladder at the posterior portion of their body develop or conclude their development in the body cavities or in subcutaneous pseudocysts in their intermediate hosts.

The development of *C. cellulosae* and *C. bovis* growing in the muscles or possibly in other organs is, in fact, very different. Therefore, the enclosure of the invaginated scolex inside the bladder may be principally of a protective nature. Both records in the literature and our findings indicate that the developing invaginated scolex and the growth of the spiral canal change the yet very little differentiated mother bladder into a larva, resembling in appearance the final form of other cysticerci. The development of this form may, however, under certain conditions, occur in larvae of a different size. Especially in *C. bovis*, this probably applies to stages which are of a very small size. In *C. bovis* and *C. cellulosae* the larva attains its definitive shape through the secondary development of the bladder.

More primordial conditions of the second phase of bladder development seem to be represented by the development of *C. cellulosae* (Fig. 11). Here, the bladder actually overgrows in a secondary process the whole anterior parenchymatous portion. A characteristic sign of this development is the differentiation of the neck between the anterior portion and the bladder. The histological proof is the histogenesis of this connecting portion. The short section between the neck and the bladder becomes so prolonged by the gradual growth of the proliferating part of the bladder that it covers the anterior portion and forms the vestibule. With it are carried into the coalescing edges of the bladder some calcareous corpuscles which are normally

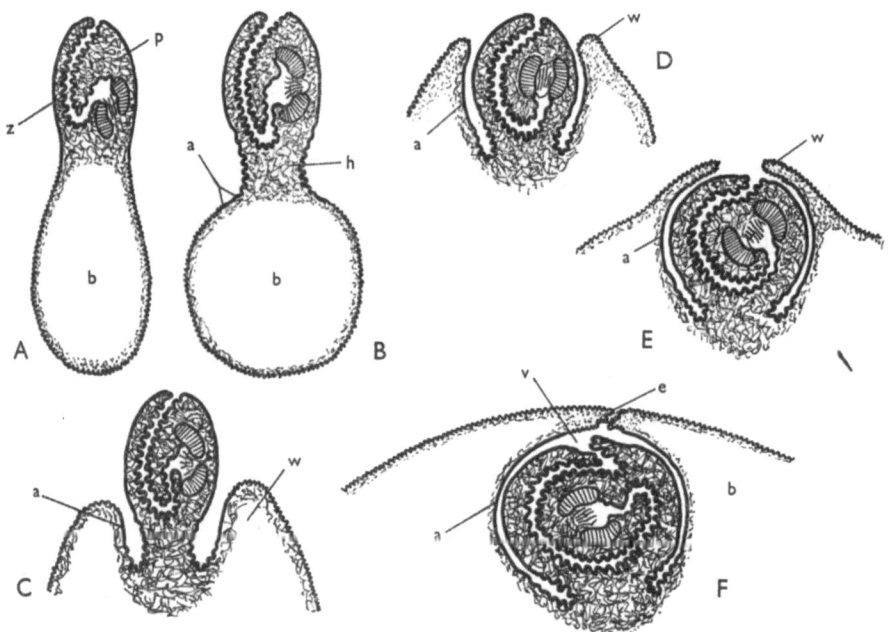

Fig. 11. Schematic illustration of the development of *C. cellulosae* from the larva with the bladder at one pole of the body (A) to the stage of the differentiating (B) and growing (C) bladder. The folds of the bladder (D) grow round the parenchymatous portion until, finally, this comes to lie in the bladder cavity (E). A small entrance canal is formed during the later growth of the bladder by a transformation of the bladder wall. The entrance canal leads into the space of the vestibule and to the primordial opening of the spiral canal (F); p — parenchymatous portion; b — bladder; a — area where the bladder wall passes into the surface of the parenchymatous portion; in fully developed forms letter "a" refers to the wall of the vestibule; w — growing folds of the bladder; v — vestibule space; e — entrance canal; z — spiral canal.

not present in the bladder wall. In the further growth of the bladder the opening of the vestibule may change into an entrance canal, which is often well-developed in overage cysticerci located in the brain.

C. bovis has no covering on its invaginated portion, the spiral canal opening directly onto the surface of the bladder and, therefore, there is no distinct border between the parenchyma and the bladder cavity. Should this cysticercus in its initial

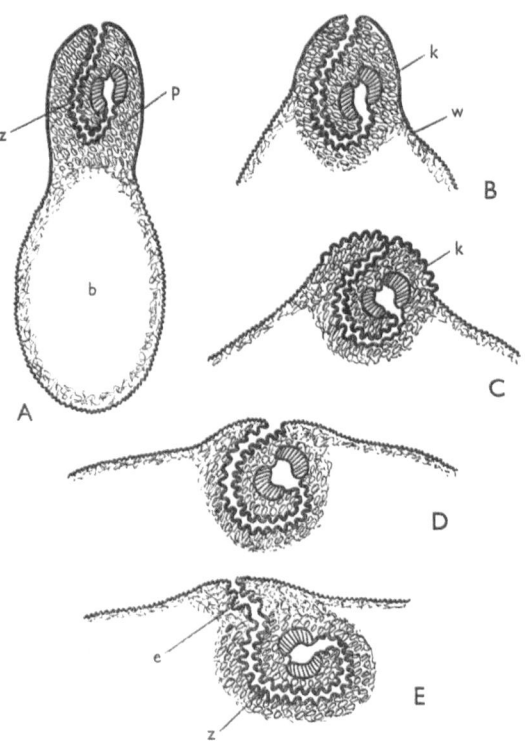

Fig. 12. Schematic illustration of the development of *C. bovis* from a larva with the bladder at one pole of its body (A). No vestibule is formed in this larva, but the parenchymatous portion splits away from the bladder wall (B); during the growth of the spiral canal its opening on the surface of the bladder becomes folded (C). When the bladder closes over the parenchymatous portion, the spiral canal opens at its surface. The lining of this spiral canal passes into the surface of the bladder (D). The opening of the spiral canal becomes prolonged during the further growth of the bladder and changes into an entrance canal. Its structure is the same as that of the surface of the bladder (E). p — parenchymatous portion; b — bladder; z — spiral canal; k — cuticle of the spiral canal and surface of the parenchymatous portion; w — transition of the cuticle into the bladder surface; e — entrance canal.

developmental stage represent a larva with an invaginated scolex, the spiral canal and the bladder being in the posterior portion, then the final form may originate from the enlarging bladder and a simultanous separation of its wall from the parenchyma containing calcareous corpuscles (Fig. 12). The separation continues up to the opening of the spiral canal. This histogenesis of *C. bovis* was confirmed by finding an example of incomplete separation and by observing two anomalous forms. When the bladder continues in its growth, an entrance canal is formed even in *C. bovis*, this, however, being the direct continuation of the spiral canal. Under certain conditions, however, for example when *C. cellulosae* becomes located in man, the parasite may develop in the same way as *C. bovis*. This was confirmed by some of our findings. After the excessive development of the entrance canal it is very difficult to reconstruct the mode of development of the brain cysticercus. There may have been some similar forms in the material of Leuckart to suggest his view of the morphogenesis of *C. cellulosae* as mentioned in the introduction to this chapter.

Another possible explanation may be the fact that sometimes in the early stage of development the invaginated scolex occupies only a small part of the original bladder cavity in larvae of 2—3 mm in diamater. This may lead to the origin of forms similar to those described by Leuckart. SCHAAF (1906) who took a critical view of some considerable shortcomings in Leuckart's descriptions, pictured similar bladders with a simple, but completely developed scolex, finding at the opening of the spiral canal various irregular folds. Also he admitted having found numerous cysticerci of irregular and variable shape and, in accord with Leuckart's concept, he considered these to be forms with a developing vestibule. In these cysticerci the anlage of the scolex measured 0·4—1 mm in diamater, but no measurements were given for the length of the bladder. In view of the size of the invaginated portion the diameter of the bladder may have been 2—6 mm. The drawings of the author suggest a proliferation of the bladder at the opening of this simple scolex-anlage. In other cysticerci of his material, however, the invaginated portion measured 4 mm in diameter and the bladder 12—14 mm in length. In appearance these were very similar to the cysticerci with a complicated spiral canal, discovered by us in the musculature of swine. Therefore, Schaaf's view that these forms originated from earlier forms by a mere further growth of the spiral canal and by an enlargement of the bladder, is subjective and unconfirmed.

A very different development occurs in the larvae of the cestode *Hydatigera taeniaeformis* (Batsch, 1786), designated *Sc. fasciolaris*, which is generally not considered to be a standard form of a cysticercus. Nevertheless the early stages of this parasite develop on the same lines although their development is considerably faster. The bladder formed by a thin wall appears very early; the scolex originates and differentiates in it in the usual invaginated position. By observing this in our own material we support de RYCKE's standpoint (1963) which rejects the view that the scolex of the strobilocercus becomes differentiated in an uninvaginated position. However, the further development of the bladder of this parasite becomes completely suppressed and attains its normal position at the end of the thin neck by further growth. The neck elongates and strobilation occurs as early as in the cyst in the liver of the intermediate host. The characteristic development of the scolex on a neck in this cysticercus is analogous to similar forms in other cysticerci, which will be discussed in a separate chapter. While in the strobilocercus the development of the bladder is suppressed, in other larval forms of cestodes, as for instance in the coenurus and the echinococcus, the bladder represents the principal portion of the larva, containing numerous scolices of simple shape. In the echinococcus the histological differentiation of the bladder becomes highly specialized by the formation of a hyaloidinic membrane. In the alveococcus the significant proliferation of the bladder confirms that in comparison with the other cysticerci these larvae attained a qualitatively different stage of development. But under extraordinary conditions such a tendency was observed also in the bladder of *C. cellulosae*, as will be discussed in the chapter on the racemose form of this cysticercus.

## 5. Histology and histochemistry of the cysticercus

Microscopic studies of cysticerci revealed two distinct basic components differing in structure: these are the surface and the parenchyma of the body and, inside the bladder, the cavity with the liquid. As previously mentioned, an early differentiation of these components was observed during the development of the oncosphere in a mother-bladder. Histologically these components represent a complex of tissues and simple organs characteristic of the whole group of platyhelminths. There are, in fact, no substantial differences between the microscopic structure of the cysticercus and that of the adult cestode except that in the latter the sexual organs develop in the parenchyma of the proglottids.

The surface of the body of a cestode is formed by a homogeneous cuticle. Views on the structure of this tegument, its layers, composition and, especially, its relationship to the so-called subcuticula have varied. The subcuticula is formed by cells which are separated from the proper cuticle by a basement layer (membrane) and particularly by a distinct layer of circular and longitudinal muscle fibres. Similar conditions occur in digenetic trematodes. Most of these studies are concerned with the adult form, but in cestodes there is hardly a difference between the surface of the scolex in the adult form and the surface of the canal leading to the invaginated scolex in the cysticercus. The structure of the surface of the bladder is, however, different and on its transition into the invaginated canal it is possible to observe the relationship of the histological structure of both surfaces. A very exact observation of these structures of the cysticercus was made by RÖSSLER (1902).

Contrary to that of the bladder wall the structure of the cuticle of the spiral canal is very distinct. It is formed by a main inner layer and a thinner superficial (outer) layer, the structure of the latter consisting sometimes of very short, parallel rods. According to our findings the main component in the cuticle is a protein; mucopolysaccharides are unevenly distributed and are more concentrated in the outer layer. The presence of mucopolysaccharides is greatly masked by the protein; this may have been the reason why WAITZ (1963) failed to obtain metachromasia with toluidine blue. This finding, however, does not furnish any reason for suggesting that acid mucopolysaccharides are not present, because positive results were obtained with alcyan blue at pH 0·2. The presence of an acid mucopolysaccharide in the cuticle of cestodes was emphasized also by MONNÉ (1959).

Because of a substantial similarity between the structure of the tegumental surface of the invaginated spiral canal of the cysticercus and the tegument of the adult cestode (Fig. 13), it is probable that their ultrastructure also is similar. Observations leading to similar findings on the ultrastructure of the tegumental surface were reported by THREADGOLD (1962) for *Dipylidium caninum*, by ROTHMAN (1963) for *Hymenolepis diminuta*, by THREADGOLD (1965) for *Proteocephalus pollanicoli*, by LUMSDEN (1966) for *Hymenolepis diminuta*, *Lacistorhynchus tenuis* and *Calliobothrium verticillatum*, by MORSETH (1966) for *Echinococcus granulosus*, *Taenia hydatigena* and *Taenia pisiformis*, by RACE et al. (1966) for *T. multiceps*. Their results, partly reviewed by LEE (1966) showed that the cuticle and the subcuticula are a special ectodermal tissue with a syncytial arrangement. The cuticle is the synplasmatic border of the distal cytoplasm without cell nuclei and the cytoplasmatic extensions maintain the continuity with the perinuclear cytoplasm, which lies in the parenchyma beneath a layer of muscle fibres. This indicates a communication with the subcuticular cells described in classic histology; but even here the transition of their distal processes into the cuticle had already been recorded by RÖSSLER (1902). The distal cytoplasm rests on a fibrous basal layer (basal zone) consisting of small fibrous filaments. This zone surrounds and separates even the individual fibres of the muscle layer, this being the finest fibrous network of the parenchyma known in classic histology as the basal membrane. Therefore, we could demonstrate it with Gomori's method for reticulin which revealed also small openings through which the cytoplasmatic continuity between the body of the subcuticular cell and the plasmatic surface is maintained. The proper proximal ultramicroscopic limiting membrane of the distal cytoplasm is attached to the muscle bundles with fine strands crossing the basal fibrous zone. The distal cytoplasm contains vesicular inclusions, dense bodies and mitochondria in its basal portion. The surface layer of the cuticle as defined in classic histology is identical with the surface projections of the distal cytoplasm. These projections although cell microvilli in nature, are of a more complicated structure and, therefore, termed microtriches. The proximal portion of the microtriches is medullated, its matrix is dispersed, finely granulated and continuous with the matrix of the distal cytoplasm. The cortex of the microtriches is more compact, the distal portion being dense, unmedullated, highly osmiophilic and tapered. Also the "pore canals", tubular formations traversing the distal cytoplasm but not forming cellular boundaries, could be demonstrated. These open directly onto the surface and connect it with the basal fibrous zone beneath the distal cytoplasm. To some writers they appeared like an evagination of this fibrous zone. In earlier electron microscopic studies this layer was called "subcuticular canal" because techniques were not yet so advanced as to detect the fine fibrils in it.

Enzymatic activity in the cuticle confirmed in histochemical studies by ROTHMAN and LEE (1963) suggests the mitochondrial nature of the cytoplasmic formation in the distal cytoplasm. The large amount of enzymes in the cuticle and the surface composed of microvilli demonstrate clearly its important resorptive function. The formation of the structural and enzymatic proteins in the subcuticular cells and their transport to the distal cytoplasm was confirmed not only cytologically by the presence of cell organoids in the perinuclear cytoplasm, but also in autoradiography (LUMS-DEN 1966).

The ultrastructure of the tegument of cestodes differs from the tegument of digenetic trematodes in the surface consisting of microvilli, the presence of pore canals and the arrangement of the mitochondria in the distal cytoplasm. In every other respect the arrangement of the body surface is the same for cestodes and trema-

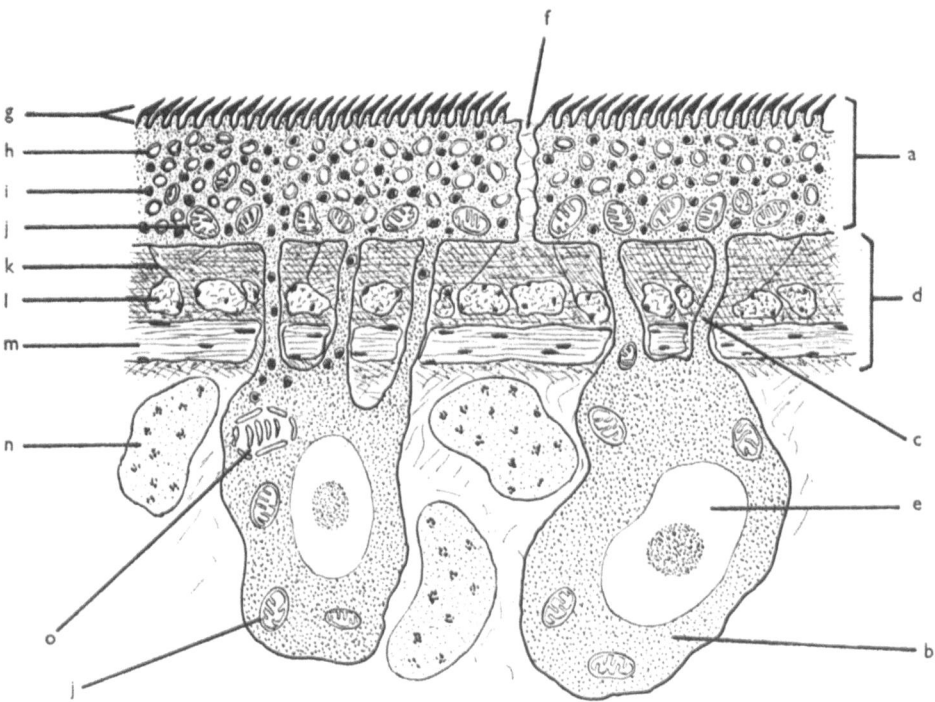

Fig. 13. Schematic illustration of the submicroscopical structure of the tegument of cestodes arranged after Threadgold and Morseth. a — distal cytoplasm; b — perinuclear cytoplasm; c — cytoplasmic extension; d — fibrous zone; e — nucleus; f — pore canal; g — microtriches; h — vesicles; i — dense bodies; j — mitochondria; k — fine connecting strands; l — circular muscle; m — longitudinal muscle; n — glycogen; o — Golgi body.

todes. This observation shows that the opinion of LOGACHEV (1955) on the exclusively mesenchymal origin of the cestode cuticle is not correct, because the surface of both groups is ectodermal in origin. Only by electron microscopic studies could this longlasting dispute on the complicated structure of the tegument be solved.

Up to the present information obtained on the tegument of the strobilar surface could not be applied analogously to the ultrastructure of the invaginated scolex. ROTHMAN (1961) found the structure of the tegument of the scolex to be very different from that of the strobila. Particularly the structure and arrangement of the microtriches were less regular and the microtriches had no cavities and resembled the distal portion of the microtriches in the surface of the strobila. Neither pore canals nor mitochondria were observed in the scolex area of *Hymenolepis diminuta*. This appearance of the tegument suggests its protective and not resorptive character. The microtriches of the segments seem to perform a double function, the medullated lower portion representing the resorptive area, while the solid distal portion serves for protection. The marked curving of their distal solid ends all in the same direction away from the main axis, indicates that when lying close together they may form a smooth protective surface. A differentiation of the microtrichal functions was suggested even by ROTHMAN (1966) who found a different location of alkalic phosphatase only on the outer membrane of the proximal portion of microtriches and a marked cholinesterase in their distal portion.

MORSETH (1967) observed in the protoscolices of the echinococcus the presence of medullated microtriches on the surface of the distal cytoplasm on the anterior portion of the scolex and even on the surface of the suckers. The posterior area of the protoscolex is covered with knoblike medullated projections with dense caps and protected by a coating of PAS-positive material. During the further development of this scolex area after its evagination these caps transform into the spike portion of the microtriches. Therefore, SMYTH et al. (1966) suggested that the surface of the protoscolex in the echinococcus could clearly function as a resorptive area. The contact with the mucosa of the gut is so close that the organism appears more like a tissue parasite than an intestinal one. This close "placental" contact is established with the aid of special rostellar glands in the scolex of the echinococcus described by SMYTH (1964) in an earlier paper. Medullated microtriches and "pore canals" were also observed by RACE et al. (1966) in the scolex of *T. multiceps*, providing more evidence of the differences among the various cestode species. These findings indicate the possibility of detecting in studies of the ultrastructure of the invaginated scolex of cysticerci, which portion of the invaginated canal persists and which portion is digested in the intestine of the definitive host. In the same way the functional activity or inactivity of the invaginated scolex may be revealed to obtain essential information on the physiology of the cysticercus in general.

WAITZ (1963) noted different PAS reactions in the tegument of larvae and adults of *Hydatigera taeniaeformis*. In the larva the reaction is more uniform in its whole cuticle; in the adult cestode the reaction is stronger and most marked in the outer cuticular layer. Although the morphology of the strobilocercus is different this may indicate that the tegument of the invaginated portion of the cysticercus becomes functionally important only after evaginating in the gut of the definitive host. The question whether it actually protects the scolex and the adjacent portion against digestion or whether it participates in the resorption of nutrient material remains to be decided.

There is little certainty about the function of the cuticular surface of the bladder wall. Characteristic of the structure of the transitional area, where the surface of the invaginated canal coalesces with the surface of the bladder, is the paucity of subcuticular cells and their shallow recession into the parenchyma. The subcuticular network of muscle fibres is also less developed and therefore, the cells lie close to the cuticle and communicate with it with their distal processes. Their numbers in the bladder wall are even less great; their shape is polygonal and irregular. Their communication with the cuticle, here much reduced in thickness, is difficult to demonstrate. The distance between the cells depends on the expansion of the bladder wall. The tension on the tissue being under the pressure of the liquid in the bladder is responsible for the special histological structure of its surface. Rössler (1902) explained this fact very clearly and proved the epithelial origin of these cells although, in view of their shape they are still considered to be of mesenchymal origin. Recently Logachev also supported this view in a number of communications. His concept (Logachev 1959) that the typical subcuticular cell layer in the cysticercus does actually not exist, is not correct. During the active growth of the bladder these cells become typically spindle-shaped and form the epithelial layer in which they divide. This cell division is amitotic.

The most typical formation in the cuticle of the bladder wall is the surface layer with the hair-like extensions, which are not cilia but a brush border. These extensions are thinner and longer than the processes of the brush border in proper resorptive cells. The cuticle itself is generally thin and forms the basis of this extension. Work on the histological structure of the bladder wall in cysticerci developing inside the tissues and organs, has not markedly progressed and little has been added to the very exact observations of earlier writers. Holz and Petzenburg (1957) suggested that the fibrilar structures under the cuticle of the bladder wall in *C. bovis* are processes of the subcuticular cells, which pass through the cuticle and continue as hair-like processes on its surface. Voge (1963) in her histological studies of *C. bovis* and *C. cellulosae* suggested considering the different length and shape of the superficial cuticular extensions as a feature differentiating their bladders. However, she found no explanation for the longer extensions in *C. bovis*. Their length seems to depend on the age of the cysticercus and on the reaction of the host tissue. The true nature of these cuticular processes can be revealed only by electron microscopy. Although the teguments of the adult cestode have been extensively examined by electron microscopy, the ultrastructure of the bladder wall of the cysticercus has been neglected so far. Waitz (1961) observed a microvillus-like surface in the larva *Hydatigera taeniaeformis*. Siddiqui (1963) on the grounds of his own electron microscopic studies contradicted the statement that the extensions run up from the basement layer of the cuticle of cysticerci to the surface. Race et al. (1965) described these formations from the bladder wall of the larva *Multiceps serialis* as proper extensions of the cuticle being medullated in one half of their length. They may possibly be homologous with the microtriches in the body surface of the adult cestode. However, the microtriches of the adults are considerably smaller and different in size and are rather column-like formations with a pointed cap. The ratio of height and width is 4 : 1 in *T. hydatigera* and *T. pisiformis*, 5 : 1 in

*Echinococcus granulosus*. Also in the adult *T. multiceps* this relationship is similar (index 7), while the microtriches of the cuticular surface of the larva of this species, the coenurus, are slender and elongated with an index of 30. In the electron microscope the tegument of the coenurus appears as a continuous, highly vacuolated layer with mitochondria in its lower half and a limiting basement membrane. However, these authors failed to observe the occurrence of subcuticular cells and their possible relationship to the cuticle as demonstrated in adult trematodes and cestodes. The cuticle of the bladder wall of the coenurus consists of a distal cytoplasm of the same composition as the cuticle of the adult forms. Perhaps the paucity of subcuticular cells in the bladder wall may have been the reason why they have not been detected and it will be most difficult to reveal their presence by electron microscopy. According to the authors mentioned above the microtriches are interconnected with fine filaments, which were not observed in the adult cestode. All these findings which are in accord with the classic histological concept on differences in the structure of the surface of the body wall in the adult cestode and in the surface of the bladder wall of the cysticercus suggest that even the function of both these surfaces may be different.

The term parenchyma, although in general use, is not very satisfactory for designating the interstitial tissue of the worms. Mesenchyme is used especially by HYMAN (1951) for the syncytial meshwork of fibres with fluid-filled spaces also containing free cells in digenetic trematodes. These mesenchyme cells can differentiate in many ways as demonstrated by CHENG and PROVENZA (1960). The variability of the types of cells in the parenchyma of digenetic trematodes highlights the relative cytological monotony of the cestode parenchyma and especially of that of cysticerci. Therefore, the knowledge obtained on the ultrastructure of the parenchyma of the liverfluke (GALLAGHER and THREADGOLD 1967) is of little help in elucidating the histological organisation of the parenchyma in cestodes.

The fundamental and practically only cell type in the parenchyma of cysticerci is a small cell with a large oval nucleus. The excessively branched cytoplasm resembles in shape the multipolar ganglionic cell of vertebrates. LOGACHEV (1958) called it the "basophilic amebocyte". These cells produce the ground substance of fine fibres and fibrils also encompassing the muscle fibres. The fibres of this complicated meshwork enter also between the subcuticular cells and form the basement layer under the cuticle, which was discussed above. The processes of the parenchymal cells are long, very branched and anastomozing. The contact between the ground substance and the cellular processes is very close, but with a suitable staining method (intravital staining with methylene blue) these cells can be differentiated from the ground substance. A fluid was demonstrated in the interstices of the meshwork of parenchymal tissue. On the inner side of the bladder of the cysticercus the parenchymal cells are closely packed and form a border separating the tissue from the fluid in the bladder cavity.

Calcareous corpuscles are very numerous in the interstices of the parenchymal meshwork of the invaginated portion (Plate V), but very scarce in the bladder wall. A detailed account of these corpuscles was given by VIRCHOW (1857). RÖSSLER (1902), finding remnants of cells on the surface of these corpules suggested that they originated from the deposition of calcium salts in the mother cell, pressing its nucleus to the periphery. YOUNG (1908) concluded that concretions are formed in the interstices of the parenchymal meshwork without a direct communication with the cells.

The calcareous corpuscles are mostly of the same size, ovoid in shape, their longer diameter measuring 18 μm, the shorter diameter 14 μm. They are composed of concentric lamellae; sometimes the surface-layer clearly differs from the median portion. Inorganic constituents of these corpuscles could be demonstrated, for example, by the staining technique of Kossa. Other methods of staining revealed also organic constituents. BRAND et al. (1960) demonstrated in the organic component of the calcareous corpuscles of *Sc. fasciolaris* a glycogen-like polysaccharide, a mucopolysaccharide, lipids and proteins. Electron microscopy revealed a lamellar structure and, in vivo, the noncrystalline state of the mineral component. SCOTT et al. (1962) found an inorganic component existing as an amorphous calcium phosphate and an amorphous complex of $Mg—Ca—CO_2$. CHOWDURY et al. (1962) demonstrated in the calcareous corpuscles even an alkalic phosphate and explained the positive Feulgen reaction as a result of the presence of remnants of the cellular nucleus, supporting thus the theory of their origin from a transformation of the parenchyma cells. Later VON BRAND et al. (1965a) confirmed the previously reported fact that the calcareous corpuscles in the various species differ mainly in the relative proportion of $Ca : Mg : P : CO_2$. In their studies of these corpuscles isolated from larval echinococci, which they collected from different localities in the world, VON BRAND et al. (1965b) found only minor differences and concluded that the differences in the composition of corpuscles from different cestode species are probably essentially species-specific. In a recent study VON BRAND et al. (1967) stated that the variation in the composition of the corpuscles is greatly dependent on the cestode species and independent of the type of host.

At present the function of the calcareous corpuscles is still obscure. BIAGI and PINA (1964) demonstrated with immunofluorescence that a positive antigen reaction is located in the calcareous corpuscles of *C. cellulosae*. DE PITA, PRATT and BIAGI (1965) tried to prepare from them an antigen of higher specific properties than the standard homogenates prepared from whole cysticerci. However, when using antigen prepared only from pure isolated calcareous corpuscles, they obtained no positive results.

The special differentiation of the parenchyma can be observed in the fibrous tissue which, in the invaginated cysticercus, forms the layer separating the surface of this portion from the bladder fluid and, after the evagination of the cysticercus, the central portion of its body. This tissue consists of numerous closely packed fibrils each with an adjoining small, spherical nucleus; the cytoplasm of these cells is almost invisible. It stains mainly as does the connective tissue of vertebrates, but its elasticity and the role played during the process of evagination indicate that it is functionally differentiated for contraction. Some thicker filaments bear the character of muscle fibres. The fibrils are too fine for detecting their inner structure on histological slides. On the fibres, however, varicosities can be observed which, in their make-up, are analogous to those found on proper muscle fibres and identified by RÖSSLER (1902) as a sign of contraction.

Even the staining properties of the differentiated muscle fibrils in the parenchyma of the cysticercus and especially in the bladder wall are often atypical for the musculature in contrast to those in the suckers. YOUNG (1908) demonstrated most convincingly that the fibres of the muscle system in the cysticercus (incorrectly designated as muscles) are formed by the cementing of the original parenchyma fibrils. The muscle fibres, branched into thick bundles composed of fine filaments, are also closely communicating with the meshwork of parenchymal fibrils and often anastomosing. In the various muscle fibres the degree of contact with the cells varies. Sometimes the cells lie relatively far from them in the parenchyma. YOUNG (1908) incorrectly called these cells myoblasts although, according to him, they are neuromuscular cells by nature. LUMSDEN and BYRAM (1967) showed in a study of the ultrastructure of the more organized muscle system in the adult cestode that the contractile portion of the muscle cells consists of a single, elongated fibre (myofibre) which is not transversely striated and contains thick and thin, parallelly arranged myofilaments. The fibres are covered with sarcolemma and surrounded by a finely filamentous tissue, which forms the stroma of larger fibril bundles. Microtubular structures cross the sarcoplasmatic masses on the periphery of the fibre.

The flame cells originating from the differentiation of the parenchymal cells, represent the beginning of the excretory system. These cells remain constantly in close contact with the parenchyma. The bundles of cilia of the flame cells protrude loosely into the capillaries. Also these, joining in collecting ducts, originate from a special transformation of other parenchymal cells. RACE et al. (1965) described the ultrastructure of the cilium in the larva *Multiceps serialis* as consisting of two central and nine peripheral fibrils. MORSETH (1967) demonstrated that the cilia are fixed to the basal plate by their proximal portion consisting of a basal body and a rootlet. Also the wall of the collecting duct is formed by the modified cytoplasm of a large cell with a nucleus. Characteristic bleblike evaginations are found on the luminal border.

The ganglia of the scolex differentiate and retain their close relationship to the parenchyma. The ganglionic cells can be demonstrated with special histological methods. In addition to the specific elements they contain also supporting parenchymal cells which are also present in the lateral nerve trunks extending along the main excretory canals of the invaginated scolex. The ultrastructure of especially the integumental sensory endings of the body wall in the echinococcus was described by MORSETH (1967). The lateral nerve trunks, according to this author, consist of large number of unmyelinated processes without a cellular sheath.

# 6. Microscopical anatomy of the cysticercus

## a) The cysticercus bladder

The cuticle, sometimes almost invisible under the microscope, is a narrow homogeneous rim generally about 0·5 µm thick. When thicker (occasionally exceeding even 1 µm) it is very refractile and sharply outlined; particularly its basal border reacts more strongly to silver staining. Histochemical reactions demonstrate neutral and acid mucopolysaccharides. The height of the distinctly visible hairlike surface processes is 1—6 µm depending on the cysticercus species. Being a cytoplasmatic formation the cuticle can be easily damaged and its absence on the bladder may indicate the onset of autolysis. Sometimes, during a dystrophy of the bladder wall, the cuticle is swollen and its columnar layout makes the processes appear longer.

The layer under the cuticle is of a granular nature and a fine fibrillary network can be detected with impregnation methods. The subcuticular muscle fibres are in some places attached to the base of the cuticle. In the bladder wall they are too loosely arranged to form a concentrated muscle system, this varying considerably in the different cysticercus species. Generally the arrangement of these fibres is circular. The layer of subcuticular cells may change even without any corresponding changes in the functional state of the bladder wall, being sometimes arranged in several rows and sometimes irregular. The nuclei mainly stain well, while the plasma is difficult to demonstrate. The height of the whole subcuticular layer in an unexpanded bladder wall is about 15 µm. The fine muscle fibres project from the cuticle downwards through the cells and, beneath this layer, actually in the parenchyma, there are also thicker muscle fibres which are mainly responsible for the contraction of the bladder. The course of the fibres and their bundles in the principle muscle system of the bladder wall is mainly longitudinal and transverse.

The thickest layer of the bladder wall is its parenchymatous portion. Its height varies considerably in relation to the state of the bladders and the age of the cysticercus, its mean values ranging from 25—30 µm. The inner surface of the wall facing the bladder cavity is formed by a loose network of fibres with an elongated cell element in their centre. In the parenchymatous portion of the bladder wall it is possible to distinguish in section two types of canals. Closer to the inner surface of the wall are situated the thin canals with a more definitely staining wall especially with Goldner's method (red). In view of their dilatation their diameter is 2·5—6 µm, exceeding in thickness even 1 µm. On tangential section it is possible to see circular, riblike supports distributed at intervals of less than 1 µm. Especially in older cysticerci a rim that stains like a collagen can be detected in the outer side of the wall. Sometimes the canals seem to be followed closely by the fibrils. Minute branches (0·5 µm in diameter) extending sideways from the thin canals are winding around them (Plate III, Fig. 1).

The second type of canal measures 15 µm and above in diameter. Their wall appears only as a sharp outline or, when the diamater of the canals is larger, it becomes almost invisible. On section they are oval, often irregular to lacunary. Mostly the canals are found in closer proximity to the surface between the layer of narrow canals and the layer of subcuticular cells. Thus the parenchymal portion of the wall clearly contains two systems of excretory canals, but in sections of bladders with a dilated canal system, the parenchymatous portion of the wall appears like a spongy system of smaller branches of the main canals interwoven with coarser and fine parenchymal tissue fibres to support the wall. The lumen of the canals of both systems depends also on the degree of dilatation of the wall.

A clearer illustration of the canal system is obtained with wholemounts of the bladder wall prepared by Jasvoin's method. They demonstrate the branching of both systems which at the crossing point of the system of larger canals nearer to the surface often appear like lacunae, measuring 30 µm and more in diameter. It can also be observed that some branches of the lower network of narrow canals communicate directly with the network above. Sometimes, particularly in younger cysticerci, it is impossible to differentiate the two types of main canals and only one network of narrower canals of a mean diameter of 6—7 µm can be detected. The main parenchymal portion is evidently formed by the fine branching of the lacunary network situated closer to the surface. The subsequent transition of this network into the finest interstices could not be traced owing to the thinness of their walls, but the existence of such communication was indicated by their dilatation and the filling of these interstices with the same granular pigment as that found in the canals of the cysticercus at the onset of dystrophy. In these wholemounts we confirmed also the presence of calcareous corpuscles dispersed throughout the bladder wall. These were more frequent around the opening of the invaginated portion of the cysticercus but even this frequency is very negligible and they can be detected only exceptionally in histological sections of the bladder wall. The cell elements in the parenchymatous portion of the wall are loosely arranged containing a spherical nucleus without a distinct cytoplasma which cannot be stained even with Jasvoin's method. The flame cells, however, appearing as the beginning of the canals of the excretory system, can be clearly demonstrated with this method.

The question of the double excretory system existing only in the cysticercus remains unsolved. We feel that its solution may offer an explanation of the function of the bladder and the metabolism of the cysticercus. Our findings are in agreement with the results of PINTNER's (1896) careful studies of the excretory system of *C. cellulosae* and *C. bovis*. Furthermore we succeeded in confirming a communication between both canal networks, which was not found by Pintner, but who could not exclude the possibility of its existence. As to the vertical communications of the more superficially situated lacunary network, which he described as sometimes extending almost to the cuticle, we consider them to be artifacts. BRAUN (1894—1900) maintained having found openings of similar formations on the surface of the cuticle in *C. crassiceps*. LOGACHEV (1958) believed that the turgor of the tissue fluid filling the canal system of the bladder wall is of mechanical importance for the tension of the wall.

b)  Microscopical anatomy of the bladder wall of *Cysticercus cellulosae*

The most typical feature of the surface of the bladder wall is the wartlike surface of the cuticle (Plate III, Fig. 1 and 2), which was noted also by VIRCHOW (1860), who compared it to a tiled pavement adding, however, that this ruggedness of the surface is in no way connected with the cell nuclei lying under the surface of the wall. LEUCKART (1879—1886) had a clear conception of these wartlike protuberances of the surface. On the basis of the first description by STEINBUCH (1801) he considered their shape and size to be a typical feature of *C. cellulosae* and although admitting the occurrence of this feature also in *C. bovis* he maintained that the protuberances in the cuticle of this cysticercus are less regular and less high. ZENKER (1882) who believed these protuberances to constitute a constant feature of the bladder wall of cysticerci doubted their specificity for *C. cellulosae*. Since those times, however, the detection of these protuberances has been considered to be the most conclusive finding in the diagnosis of the cysticercus during pathological examination. According to TRELLES et al. (1952) their remarkable height and slim shape is typical of the racemose cyst of a cerebral cysticercus. We found that the wartlike surface of the cuticle of the bladder wall of the cysticercus is related to its functional state and is caused by the presence of special groups of muscle fibres. In *C. cellulosae* their make-up and occurrence is so typical that their contraction causing the wartlike surface has always been considered to be a typical feature.

In all specimens of *C. cellulosae* in muscle cysticercosis, in cerebral cysticercosis of man and in the racemose form, the surface of the bladder wall may be either rugate or smooth in appearance. On serial sections of the whole parasite we often observed part of the bladder to be smooth, part of it rugate and, in some places, intermediate between rugate and smooth. The height of the wartlike protuberances varied from 15—22 µm, their width at the basis from 27—38 µm, the index of height to width was 0·60. In places where these protuberances were particularly marked and, in the racemose cysticercus with a rugate cuticle, their width was 15—27 µm with an index 0·90. The height of the rim of cuticular, hairlike extensions ranged in *C. cellulosae* from less than 1 µm to 2·5 µm. When protuberances were present the subcuticular cell layer was concurrent and the wartlike protuberances were formed only by the granular component of the subcuticular layer with its fibrillar network and short muscle fibres traversing in almost stellar fashion (Plate XXII, Fig. 4). In an expanded wall these muscle groups were stretched and appeared like very elongated, lunate formations with raised centres, disturbing the regular coherence of the subcuticular cell layer. The length of these stretched muscles averaged about 60 μm throughout the groups. Therefore, in wholemounts representing the complete bladder wall, the subcuticular cell layer of a cuticle with a wartlike surface appeared as a layer of evenly distributed nuclei (Plate IV, Fig. 4). In the expanded wall the nuclei seemed to be pressed into stripes forming a network of empty, almost circular areas of the diameter previously indicated (Plate IV, Fig. 6). Further evidence of the functional changes in the bladder wall was the changing number of subcuticular cells. On a 0·06 mm long wall with a rugate surface the number of cells was 11 compared with only 6—7 cells on the same length of expanded wall surface. The finding of stretched muscles is very characteristic of *C. cellulosae* and they were observed in all cases of cysticercosis even if the wartlike surface of the cuticle of the parasite's bladder could not be detected. It has to be mentioned that this rugate surface is in no way connected with the folds in the bladder wall originating from contractions of the main muscle system, because these derange completely the uniform pattern of the protuberances. The staining character of the special subcuticular fibres is often identical with that of the muscle fibres, so that in some instances it may be difficult to distinguish in the bladder wall connective tissue fibres from the muscle fibres by staining methods. This may evidently be connected with the still little advanced differentiation of the muscle fibres in the bladder wall of the cysticercus. It is remarkable that in larvae which are starting to autolyse, these subcuticular muscle fibres are noticeably swollen and stain most characteristically like musculature (Plate XXII, Fig. 3).

The typical appearance of these special subcuticular muscles is particularly characteristic in muscles which are relaxed in a bladder wall which is not expanded. At this stage, when there may be an indication of the wartlike surface or when the surface is smooth, the diameter of the individual muscle groups corresponds with the base of the protuberances or may be even slightly larger (40—50 μm). The fibres, however, are inserted in looplike fashion to the cuticle.

This appearance of the fibres is most striking in bladders at the onset of growth. (Plate XXII, Fig. 1 and 2). At this time, relatively thick-walled folds of growth originate on the bladder, inside which especially the subcuticular cells start to reproduce, forming a marked proliferation zone of cells which attains a height of up to 15 μm. In it, the basophilic plasma is very distinct. Many cells are multinucleated and divide by amitosis. In some instances, however, even a fragmentation of the nuclei has been observed. In this respect these cells are very similar to the proliferating subcuticular zone of growth in the scolex portion of the parasite. In places where the wall has just started to grow it becomes attenuated and the cell layer at the site of transition from the folds splits into groups of 4—6 nuclei under the insertions of the muscles, the distance between them being 40 − 50 μm. In places where growth is most marked there are 5—6 cells on 0·06 mm of wall length, hence less than in the expanded wall. As was observed during the overgrowing of the scolex portion of *C. cellulosae*, the signs of growth are particularly marked at the peak of the fold. The wall is very attenuated, its structure indistinct, the distance between the small groups of cells is 35—45 µm, at the peak of the fold even 70—80 µm.

The aging of the bladder wall of *C. cellulosae* was studied in developed cerebral forms. The wall is mostly very thick, this thickness ranging from 50—180 µm. The parenchymatous portion is of a typically hyaline appearance. The subcuticular muscles are very flattened, but their lunar shape can be distinguished (Plate XXII, Fig. 5) particularly from the fact that these sites are not silver staining with Gomori's technique. However, silver staining with this method gives best results when the reticular skeleton of the wall has started to increase in the process of aging, this ensuring the identification of even necrotic bladder walls. Often, the onset of necrotic and autolytic changes disturbing the structure of the wall is followed by excessive contraction of the cuticular surface; the initial autolysis makes the subcuticular muscles fuse into balls and causes disintegrating changes in the ducts.

LEUCKART (1879—1886) drew attention to the limited development of the muscle network under the cuticle of the bladder in comparison with the scolex portion in *C. cellulosae*. He considered the fine branching of the muscle fibres intermixing and at the same time coalescing with the fibrillar layer under the cuticle to be a most remarkable feature. Our demonstration of the special muscle fibres in this zone fully supports his idea that the elucidation of the relationship and connection of this branching muscle network with the cuticle may reveal the reason for the wartlike surface of the cuticle in this cysticercus. The complete explanation of this question in other cysticerci examined is frustrated by difficulties in staining these fine muscle fibres, this making it impossible to differentiate them from the branching network of fibres of a reticular nature. TRELLES et al. (1952) stained these typical subcuticular muscles of *C. cellulosae* in a racemose form of cerebral cysticercus by Hortega's method with ammoniacal silver impregnation. They believed them to constitute the terminal branching of fibrils and canals without recognizing their relationship to the wartlike surface of the cuticle in spite of the fact that they found them in a less marked form also in the relatively smooth wall of *C. cellulosae* from swine.

## c) Microscopical anatomy of the bladder wall of *Cysticercus bovis*

The bladders of *C. bovis* when fixed with the surrounding tissue, were always smooth without protuberances on their surface both in live and dead specimens. In live bladder fixed after being recovered from the tissue, the protuberated surface (covered with protuberances) of the wall which is clearly visible in live cysticerci was retained in varying degree. The shagreen appearance of the surface is very typical and remains unchanged even during the contractions of the bladder resembling peristaltic waves. In sections the protuberances appear like coarse formations of the cuticle and the subcuticular cell layer. The size of the protuberances is less uniform than in the wartlike formations in the cuticle of *C. cellulosae* (Plate III, Fig. 3). In *C. bovis* these are not protuberances of the cuticle and of the fibrillar layer underneath it, but superficial formations of the bladder wall. Several layers of densely packed subcuticular cells constitute the base of each fold, while in the upper margin they are arranged only in a single row. Therefore, (Plate IV, Fig. 5) the layer of subcuticular cells in a smooth bladder wall appears in wholemounts like an area containing evenly distributed nuclei. When the wall surface is protuberated the nuclei of these cells in the protuberances can be focussed in several layers under the microscope; along their borders we often noticed light strips (Plate IV, Fig. 3) of contracted muscle fibres in which nuclei of subcuticular cells could not be shown. In agreement with this the insertions of muscle fibres into the cuticle as seen on the sections were arranged largely in strips of various length and the fibres, mostly projecting through the cell layer, continued under it. The protuberated surface of the bladder wall in *C. bovis* is thus originating from the contraction of a system of traversing strips of muscle fibres, this being responsible for the arching of the bladder surface mainly in sites which are not crossed by muscle fibres. Especially after fixation, the dimensions of these protuberances are less uniform and their height varies from 23—24 μm with several peaks and bases of different size ranging from 50 to 70 μm, but always considerably larger than in *C. cellulosae*. Also the ratio of their average height to width being 0·40 indicates their rather flat shape. The height of the hairlike extensions on the surface of the cuticle ranges from 3—6 μm and is greater than in *C. cellulosae*.


d)   Scolex portion of the cysticercus

The parenchymatous portion of the cysticercus consists of the invaginated scolex with the hooks and the suckers and of the canal either spirally coiled or only meandering with a folded wall leading to the bladder surface. This relatively massive portion is not covered with a special tissue layer at the side facing the bladder cavity, being made up of the parenchyma with its complicated system of interstices in the tissue and of excretory canals. The parenchyma of the invaginated portion of the parasite contains a large amount of glycogen persisting until late into advanced autolysis.

The surface of the spiral canal terminating in a cavity with the suckers and the rostellum is of a similar structure to that of the bladder surface. The subcuticular layer of the recessed epithelium, however, is of a more noteworthy appearance consisting of a layer of elongate, densely packed cells located under the superficial cuticle. The cells constitute the main component of this subcuticular zone. The bottom border of the cuticle is formed mainly by a layer of marked muscle fibres traversing at right angles and forming a thick, homogeneous, regular network (Plate XXIII, Fig. 3). This is enclosed in the ground substance of fine fibrillar material, staining like connective tissue and colouring green with Goldner's method. This substance is particularly dense on the floor of the cuticle forming the basal layer of its bottom border. After silver staining with Gomori's method this layer becomes very marked and it is then possible to demonstrate in it the regularly distributed apertures of equal size, measuring markedly less than 1 μm (Plate XXIII, Fig. 4). The proper, relatively high homogeneous cuticle (15—18 μm) is of a fine, granular appearance, in *C. cellulosae* often with deeper grooves (Plate XXIII, Fig. 1). A rim of fine projections on its surface can be discovered only occasionally and very indistinctly, appearing generally as a thin, superficial border-layer. In view of the fact that it stains with Goldner's method and with the method after Hale, the proper cuticle may be characterized as a complex of mucopolysaccharides and proteins (Plate XXIII, Fig. 2). It even stains, though feebly, with Sudan black B. The main amino acid to be detected was tryptophane. Numerous calcareous corpuscles were revealed mainly in the parenchymal tissue of the folds in the spiral canal under the cuticle and the subcuticular layer (Plate V). The number of these corpuscles varies in the different cysticerci. The difference between the invaginated scolex of *C. cellulosae* enclosed in a special replicate of the bladder wall (the "vestibule", see p. 30) and the invaginated scolex of *C. bovis* projecting directly into the bladder cavity, is also reflected in the microscopical structure of both these portions.

The invaginated scolex of *C. bovis* with its canal opening directly on the bladder surface, is more expanded and the wall of the canal is also less deeply folded (Plate XXI, Fig. 1 and 2). The parallely arranged fibrous tissue originating from the so-called receptaculum and constituting the axial body in the evaginated scolex, is spread out in a layer on the surface of the invaginated formation. It forms the inner surface of the parenchymatous portion in the region where it faces the bladder cavity. The fibrous layer is sharply bordered off from the parenchyma of the folds of the invaginated canal which, in contrast to the fibrous layer, is packed with calcarous corpuscles. Along this demarcation line proceeds the excretory system of the scolex, originating from a coalescence of both types of canals of the bladder wall. These excretory canals of the bladder wall coalesce at the opening of the spiral canal and thus form the typical lateral canals which meander along the above mentioned demarcation line up to the rostellum of the invaginated scolex. Along this line runs also a distinct layer of muscle fibres. These are more numerous and smaller in diameter in the rostellar region, while more marked and less numerous the closer they come to the opening of the invaginated canal. Round this opening they blend with the main muscle system of the bladder wall, but some of them continue until they reach the cuticle. Their contraction accounts for the folds in the bladder wall characteristically found round the opening of the canal. These are often seen in sections. This network of muscle fibres plays an important role in the process of scolex evagination, which results in the elasticity of the fibrous tissue following release of internal tension.

In *C. cellulosae*, the whole inner formation is more compressed, the invaginated canal being spirally coiled for lack of space. Its surface is deeply folded and the grooves in the cuticle, so typical for this species are, in fact, only the manifestation of a second-ary folding of the cuticle on the surface of the main folds. (Therefore, these folds are most exceptional in the outermost portion of the canal in *C. bovis*). Also the basal layer under the cuticle is greatly thickened by compression under the folds of the cuticle, while it is almost invisible under the groove. The fibrous tissue is very ex-panded and extends along the outer side of the spiral canal ending under the suckers and the rostellum. It is contiguous with the bladder cavity only at the place where it is thickest, resembling a parenchymal, knob-like formation which connects the invaginated scolex with the wall of the vestibule. Except for the results of the great compression of the spiral canal there are no significant differences in the composition of this portion of these two cysticerci.

## 7.   Morphology of the parasite in cysticercosis of man

The structure of the cysticercus in the brain of man is sometimes the same as that of the typical bladder in the muscle of swine, but mostly there are striking differences in the tissues of the parenchymatous portion with the invaginated scolex, these being more markedly developed. They form partly the thick outer wall sur-rounding the whole parenchymatous portion of the cysticercus, partly the long entrance canal of this portion. The spiral canal leading from the rostellum and the suckers of the invaginated scolex, opens between the folds and the blind appendages at the end of this entrance canal, which only then, usually directly, proceeds to the bladder surface (Fig. 14). Fully developed bladders having reached advanced age and the limit of their vitality, are usually of oval shape, measuring up to 25 mm in length and up to 15 mm in width. The length of the invaginated portion of the cysticercus is 5 mm and even more (Plate VI, Fig. 3).

The histological structure of the spiral canal leading to the rostellum and the suckers of the invaginated scolex, is practically the same as that of the bladder from swine with the exception of some slight differences in the structure of the folds and curves round its opening into the entrance canal and in the initial part of this canal. The cuticle is less high, ungrooved, the cells in the subcuticular layer are not elongated but rather spherical in shape. There are more interstices and lacunae but less calcareous corpuscles in the parenchyma. The excretory canals and their branches are situated directly in the folds and often even the opening of large canals can be discovered on the surface of the fold, into which the homogeneous cuticle, reduced in thickness, can project (Plate VI, Fig. 1).

Completely different is the structure of the entrance canal connecting the invaginated scolex with the bladder surface. In all cysticerci recovered from man and especially in those from the brain of man this portion was enormously developed and its volume exceeded even the proper scolex portion. Its wall was deeply folded, the layer of the homogeneous cuticle was low and often bearing a typical rim of hair-like projections (Plate VI, Fig. 2). The basal layer of connective tissue nature situated under the cuticle was completely changed. It was thick, consisting of fibres first pulpy, later homogeneous, but containing a network of the same unchanged muscle

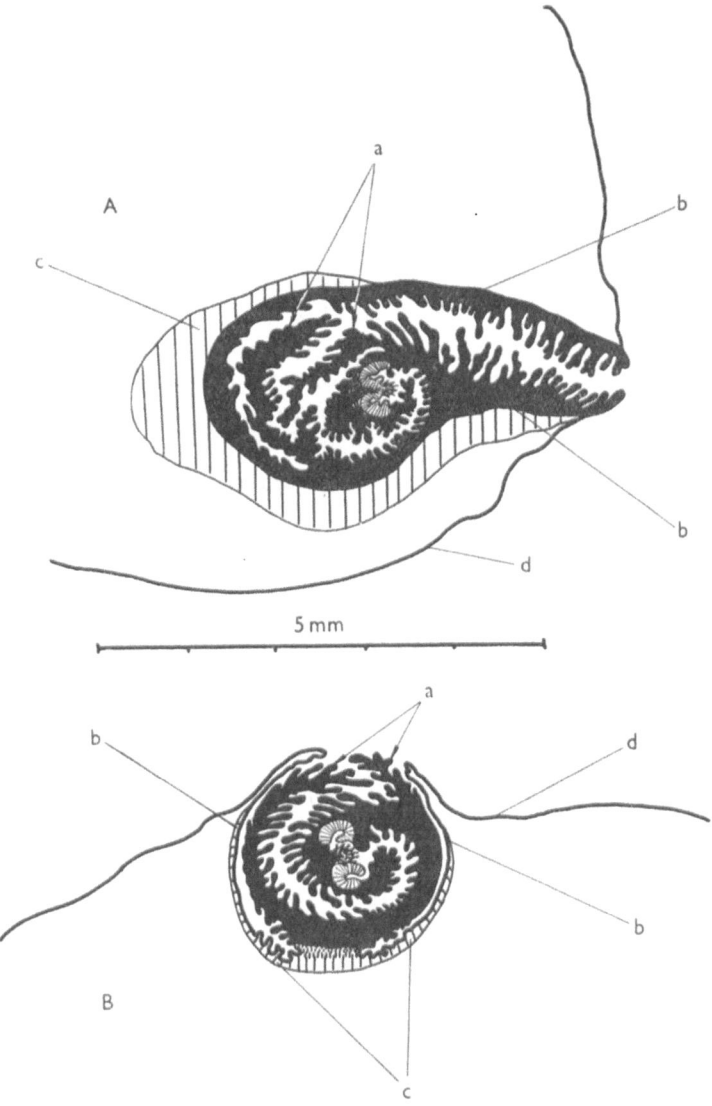

Fig. 14. Schematic comparison of the parenchymatous portion in the cerebral form of *C. cellulosae* (A) with the parenchymatous portion of this cysticercus in the muscles of swine (B). a — folds limiting the opening of the spiral canal; b — the wall of the vestibule closer to the surface of the bladder in (B) is homologous with the wall of the entrance canal in (A); c — the wall of the vestibule passing into the parenchymatous knoblike formation in (B) is homologous with the enormous amount of tissue round the main portion of the cerebral cysticercus; d — bladder wall.

fibres as those in the spiral canal. The layer was interspersed with a branching arrangement of the finest excretory canals. These were easily demonstrable when filled with a substance of presumably proteinic nature, staining blue with Mallory's haematoxylin. However, the border between this layer and the cuticle could no longer be impregnated with silver. Also the subcuticular layer of the cell elements was very discontinuous, the parenchyma was loose and formed by a tangle of fibres, lacunae and canals with a marked wall of their own and lumina of different widths. Their main branches were concentrated near the surface of the wall facing the bladder cavity and extending towards the surface of the folds. No calcareous corpuscles were discovered in this portion. Thus the surface of this entrance canal leading to the proper invaginated portion is very similar to the surface of the bladder wall. The parenchymal portion of the wall was relatively thick and often relatively large lobes of loosely arranged tissue without cell elements adjoined this wall (Plate VI, Fig. 4). In most cysticerci, these parts showed signs of dystrophy, thus being the first section of the parasite's body to succumb to autolysis during its degeneration. The entrance canal of many cerebral cysticerci was so enormous and often enlarged at its blind termination that it was almost impossible to detect the invaginated scolex among the folds.

In muscle cysticercosis of man, the appearance of the parasite was the same as that of *C. cellulosae* in swine. Only in very old cysticerci did we observe similar changes to occur as in the cerebral form.

## 8. Morphogenesis of *Cysticercus cellulosae* when localized in the brain

We succeeded in confirming the relationship between the typical cysticercus of swine and the characteristic appearance of the brain cysticercus in a number of transitional forms developing during the protracted course of the disease and the continuing growth of the cysticerci. In some of the forms the vestibule round the parenchymatous portion was still the same as in the cysticercus from swine, only its opening on the surface of the bladder was no longer simple but formed a short canal with a folded wall (Fig. 15). In another form we observed a shortening of the slit between the wall of the vestibule and the parenchymatous portion with the invaginated scolex, whereby the spiral canal continued its growth and increased in bulk. In a number of transitional forms in which the vestibule was no longer separated, we discovered the developing entrance canal in its various developmental stages (Fig. 16). Here, it was possible to demonstrate histologically the progressing differentiation mainly with Giemsa staining (Plate XXIII, Fig. 5). The border line between the cuticle of the spiral canal leading to the scolex and the transitional part leading to the entrance canal was particularly distinct. The cuticle of the spiral canal was high and typically grooved. With further differentiation using Giemsa it became rose coloured, while the colour of the narrower, smooth cuticle was still bright blue. The transitional part of these forms was relatively large and hairlike extensions were present on the surface of the cuticle, while the entrance canal was not yet so much developed. Also the glycogen content of the tissues was different, its high concentration being retained only close to the invaginated scolex. It was substantially lower in the newly formed portions.

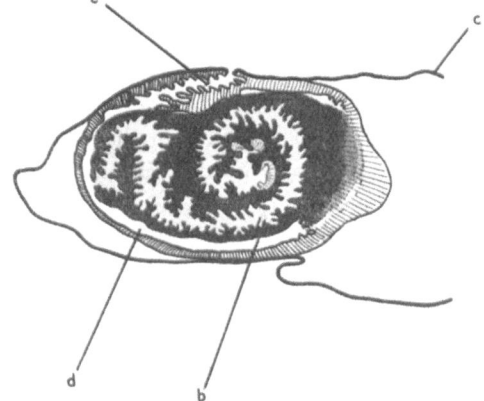

Fig. 15. Cerebral form of *C. cellulosae* with the first indication of a developing entrance canal leading into the space of the vestibule, which surrounds the highly developed spiral canal; b — spiral canal; c — bladder wall; d — space of the vestibule; e — entrance canal.

The abnormal size of the bladder and the different microscopical anatomy of this form are related to the localization of the cysticercus in the brain or in its meninges. Of primary importance is its undisturbed growth in the loose tissues of the central nervous system as compared with the growth in the muscles. The brain

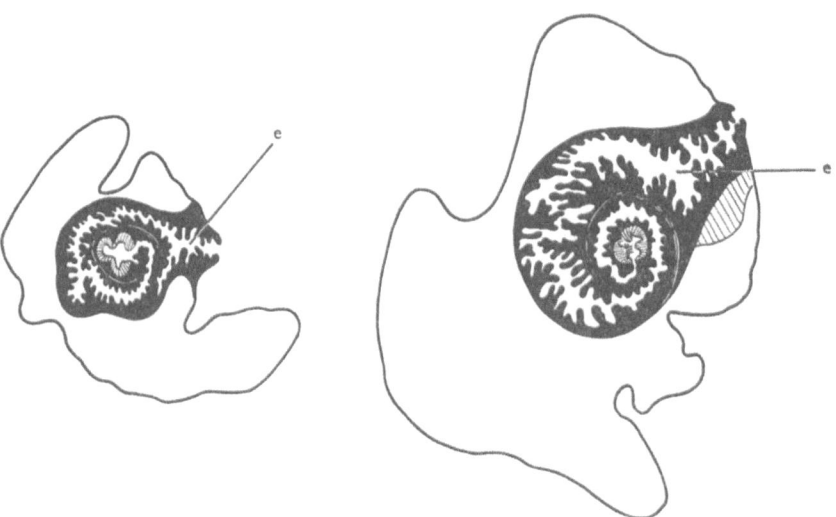

Fig. 16. Scheme of two cerebral cysticerci in which the originating entrance canal (e) passes undisturbed into the spiral canal.

*61*

chambres offer the best conditions for growth and there the parasite, lying freely, attains its largest size. The influence of location on the morphology of the parasite was also confirmed by an observation in a generalized cysticercosis; the bladders recovered from the diaphragm were of the same elongate shape as those in the muscul-ature of swine, while the bladders from the cerebellum were larger, oval and lobate. A similar influence of location on the shape of the bladder was also observed by KHE-LIMSKY (1963), whereby the histological structure was the same in the cysticercus from the musculature and that from the cerebellum. This is in keeping with the ob-servations by KITAOKA (1962), who found a similar structure of the wall in the cysticercus from the brain and in that from the musculature.

The second important factor influencing the morphology of the cerebral cysticercus is advanced age. Being located in the brain of man the cysticerci dissociate themselves from their normal life cycle and, as long as their presence in the host does not endanger his existence, they continue to grow as larvae to the end of their life. The zone of growth of the scolex is terminal and the growth of the spiral canal continuously increases its distance from the bladder wall. The opening of this canal on the bladder surface is a typical morphological feature of the cysticercus. It persists even during the exuberant growth of the bladder in that its wall growing on its whole periphery, prolongs the spiral canal by its proliferation like an entrance canal at the site of its opening.

In this very simple way the entrance canal is formed in the average *C. bovis.* In *C. cellulosae* growing in the brain, the vestibule and the characteristic outer wall of the parenchymatous portion are reduced by the formation of the entrance canal. This is characteristic for this cysticercus species and was confirmed by our findings of transitional forms. However, during the abnormal development of a young larva under unusual conditions, the formation of the vestibule is not a necessity with this species. In overage forms of *C. cellulosae* with an enormous entrance canal it is not possible to determine their mode of development.

The entrance canal, a characteristic feature of the cerebral form of *C. cellulosae,* was figured but not described by TRELLES (1952). Also VOGE (1963) did not evaluate this canal, perhaps because her comparative material was scarce or because she did not use serial sections. However, she observed the histological difference between the bladder and the invaginated portion of the bladder, calling the first the "outer tissue", the latter the "inner tissue".


## 9.   The nature of the racemose form in cerebral cysticercosis

The lobate and branched form of the cerebral cysticercus localized predomi-nantly at the base of the brain is a rare finding (Fig. 17). VIRCHOW (1860) first drew attention to the existence of some remarkable formations at the base of the brain.

With great precision he described almost all significant characters: the structure consisting of bladders of various sizes forming a single grapelike body; the fine ducts and stalks connecting all groups of bladders; the close adherence to vessels without coalescing either with them or with the tissues of the leptomeninges. Moreover, he also noticed the striking similarity with the hydatid mole and the characteristic shagreen look of the bladder surface. Although he recorded in one of his observa-

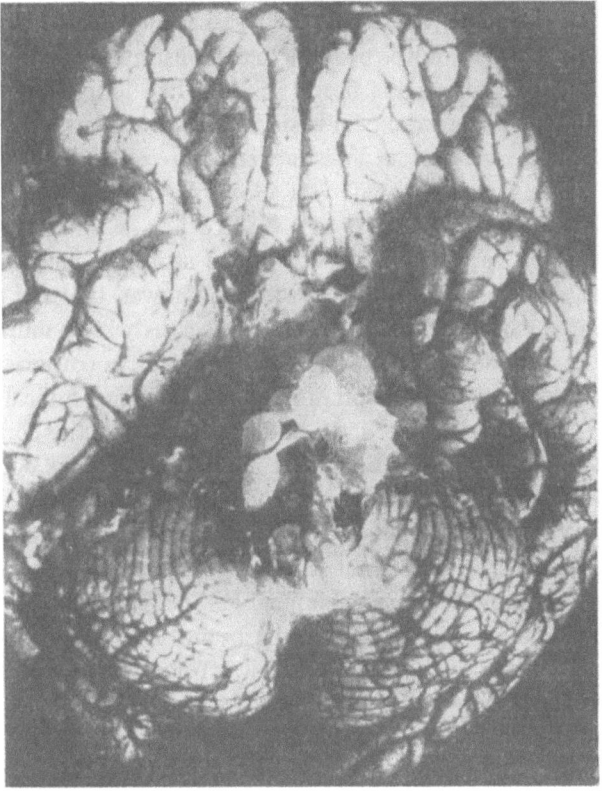

Fig. 17. Bladderlike structure of the racemose cysticercus at the base of the brain. Reproduction of an illustration by Prof. Gruber in the textbook Henke - Lubarsch.

tions the finding of a dead and calcified cysticercus in the brain, he had certain doubts about the parasitic origin of these formations.

The parasitic origin of these bladders was confirmed by ZENKER (1882) who called them *C. racemosus*. But even today there are certain aspects of their origin and occurrence which need elucidation. During recent years, the identity of this cysticercus species has been widely discussed in connection with the confirmed finding of *Coenurus cerebralis* in man.

In our observation we examined the almost complete material from an abnormal racemose form of cerebral cysticercosis at an advanced stage of resorption. The intact parts of the membrane showed the typical structure of the bladder wall of the cysticercus. In its folds the parenchymal layer was relatively thick and typically spongy and contained dispersed cell nuclei. The surface of the membrane was undulated. On the surface of the cuticle did we observe a rim of hairlike projections (Plate VII, Fig. 2). The layer of subcuticular cells was often interrupted. In places where the membrane formed cystic bodies, the wall was very attenuated and its surface was smooth (Plate VII, Fig. 1). Under the cuticle, especially in places where the surface was of a wartlike appearance, it was possible to demonstrate with Mallory's phospho-tungstic haematoxylin short muscle fibres receding like loops from their cuticular insertions. Staining with haematoxylin-eosin and with Giemsa's method revealed crescent-shaped, minute areas of an indistinct structure even under the cuticle of an expanded wall. These, when treated with Gomori's method for reticular fibres, remained unstained.

The examination of a necrotic focus in the septum pellucidum (Plate VIII, Fig. 1) by means of series of histological sections showed that the formation concerned was the large, shrivelled bladder of a cysticercus with a multifold wall. The whole formation was situated in the rostral part of the sulcus corporis callosi. During its growth it was pressing into the septum pellucidum causing a local atrophy of the cortex. Further to the caudal side, it was still delimited by the cortex, which had become attenuated. It was also possible to demonstrate the direct connection of this shrivelled bladder with the mass of cystic formations of the parasitic membrane, which continued from there through the fissura interhemispherica to the base of the brain enveloping both a. cerebralis anterior and also the a. communicans anterior. Round this artery the bundle of parasitic bladders merged with similar formations in the thickened meninges at the base of the brain. The parenchymatous portion of the cysticercus with the invaginated scolex was found neither in the focus of the shrivelled large bladder nor in the other foci with a parasitic membrane; neither were hooks found in the encapsulating tissue.

We determined our finding as a large bladder of a brain cysticercus which had started to grow in the sulcus corporis callosi under the septum pellucidum and degenerated some time later, while its bladder wall had continued to proliferate until it had reached the base of the brain as a typical *Cysticercus racemosus*. Its scolex was not found. In spite of the advanced necrosis and autolysis of the parasite we still observed in some sections all histological characters of the proliferating bladder wall of the cysticercus (Plate VIII, Fig. 2).

Another of our observations included some important and exceptional material. The complete encysted body removed by operation — a grapelike formation — constisted of differently sized bladders (Plate IX). Some of them were spherical with a thin wall and a uniform surface; some were lobate and irregular in shape with branches and branching buds projecting from some lobes (Plate XXIV, Fig. 1). These mostly solid buds were formed by the typical parenchyma of the bladder wall of the cysticercus interwoven with a system of excretory canals and slits, in which the origin of the lumen could be observed. The surface of all formations was identical with the characteristic surface of the bladder of the cysticercus with hairlike projections on the cuticle and a layer of subcuticular cells. The surface was generally smooth and expanded and even under the cuticle of the buds and their branches it was possible to note the expanded, characteristic, subcuticular muscles (Plate XXIV, Fig. 2). The cuticle of some bladders, not being enclosed in the granulation tissue, was sometimes of the wartlike appearance which is typical of *C. cellulosae*. The granulation tissue was most abundant and most infiltrated in the areas with a complicated network of bladders and branching buds, whole parts of it had become necrotic and necrosis was also spreading to the surrounding encapsulation tissue. In these parts it was possible to see all grades of a resorbing giant cell reaction.

This material was found to represent a large, partly encapsulated formation made up of a most divergent and proliferating conglomeration of cysticercus bladders which were highly necrotic and at the stage of resorption.

In material from an earlier published observation (KARPÍŠEK, VALACH 1952) which we examined anew, we even demonstrated in the bladder walls of this typical racemose cysticercus a histological structure characteristic of the bladder of *C. cellulosae* (Plate X).

Thus we discovered the process of growth of the racemose cysticercus and the proliferation of its bladder wall in all our observations. Even ZENKER (1882) failed to observe this in his monograph which is considered to be the most complete analysis of this problem up to the present. On the grounds of 16 observations, he drew attention mainly to variations in the shape of the parasite known as *Cysticercus racemosus*, distinguishing a number of formations: the simple lobate bladders; several communicating bladders; the acinous form consisting of a single cluster of secondary, sometimes pedunculate, cysts attached to the original bladder and, finally, the proper grapelike body with its complicated system of branched bladders attaining a length of 20 cm and more, this being the only type fully in keeping with the term *Cysticercus racemosus*. This variety of shapes, also described by STUCH-LÍK (1928) from a solitary observation, supplies evidence about the various stages of the further proliferation of the cysticercus bladder. The active growth of the bladder wall was confirmed by our first observation, but indisputable proof through histological confirmation of the complete agreement with the proliferation of the bladder observed in the young cysticercal stages was obtained in our second observation. Until the present, no similar case of such intensive growth of the brain cysticercus has been described in the literature.

In a fine preparation Zenker succeeded in proving communications in even the most intricately branched racemose cysts. Also KOCHER (1911) demonstrated the delicate communications in the individual parts of the cysticercus. These connections may become damaged not only by less careful preparation, but also by the onset of tissue reaction. Therefore, it is noteworthy that in most of the observations of the last century reviewed by Zenker, the large, racemose forms were not encapsulated. At that time, this was considered to be one of the characteristic features of *C. racemosus*. Only the standard forms, being slightly lobate, less large and less articulate were encapsulated. All later observations of the racemose cysticercus were discovered at an advanced stage of resorptive reaction (e.g. MENNICKE 1897, BERLINGER 1930 a.o.). TRELLES (1961) demonstrated as a typical example of a racemose cysticercus the marked thickening of the leptomeninges at the base of the brain, which covered all finer structures. We found a similar picture in our observations. Naturally, at the stage of resorption, it is impossible to demonstrate any communications among the remnants of the racemose cysticercus.

Some earlier authors believed that the absence of the fibrous capsule was responsible for the proliferation of the bladder spreading widely in the subarachnoid cavity at the base of the brain. In examining a cerebral cysticercosis we found completely free parasites under the leptomeninges in a groove at the side of the brain stem at a stage of early degeneration, but their shrivelling bladder was still of a normal size. This shows that the absence of tissue reaction is not responsible for the transformation of the cysticercus into the racemose form. As shown by our own and some other observations the resorptive reaction starts in this form at the time when the parasite is degenerating, this being the same in a standard cerebral cysticercosis. The picture of a severe, chronic, basilar meningitis and of a chronic hydrocephalus accompanying this infection is conditioned by the location of the racemose cysticercus.

The unimpeded growth of the cysticercus in the subarachnoid spaces at the base of the brain, during which the parasite can grow even retroversely into the brain ventricles (especially into the 4th ventricle) and the bladder growing round the vessels and entering the preformed slits is one of the factors which Zenker believed to be responsible for the typical lobate appearance of this cysticercus. However, there is clear evidence from our and other observations that the growing bladder itself participates in the shaping of the racemose cysticercus by forming buds and intricately branched projections. Often, a connection was found between a larger, but generally simple cyst in one part of the brain and the racemose formation at the base of the brain, similar to that demonstrated in our observation. Sometimes, the simultaneous occurrence of a racemose cysticercus with normal cysticerci was recorded from the brain of a patient (also by HAŠKOVEC 1929 and HENNER et al. 1946). On the grounds of these findings and supported by the observation of the shagreen surface of their membranes, which is typical for the bladder of the cysticercus, Zenker based his statement about the cysticercal origin of even widely branched cysts. Later he found in one of his observations of a racemose cysticercus even the scolex and hooks of the *C. cellulosae* type but, noticing signs of degeneration also in this scolex Zenker concluded that the proliferation of the bladder into such bizzare forms may start only after the degeneration of the scolex or, if no scolex has been developed. The relationship of scolices with the racemose form described by MARCHAND (1879), was not supported by sufficient evidence.

It is most difficult to identify correctly the parasite species without finding its scolex. Therefore, some authors believed that these racemose parasitic cysts at the base of the brain may cause coenurosis in man. This question is analyzed in the chapter discussing the differential diagnosis of various cysticerci in man.

## 10. Morphology and origin of invaginated cysticerci with an outgrown scolex

LEUCKART (1879—1886) explained the development of the scolex in his studies. He demonstrated that in the invaginated canal first the suckers and then, at its very end, the rostellum can be discovered. By contrast some earlier authors maintained that they had observed first the elevated rostellum situated at the end of the canal and then, below it, the suckers, in the same sequence as found on the scolex of the adult cestode. Leuckart believed these to be artifacts caused by fixation. MONIEZ (1880) observed in *C. pisiformis* scolices in normal positions arising on necks of varying length from the end of this canal sometimes extending right to the opening on the surface of the cysticercus. Probably because he had very little material Moniez imagined erronously that the development of the scolex involved a process in which the protuberance arising from the end of the invaginated canal continued to grow and, subsequently, formed the origin of the suckers and the rostellum. On the basis of his very extensive material Leuckart demonstrated without difficulty that the organs of the scolex differentiate from its wall at the end of the invaginated canal and that, during its morphogenesis, the whole scolex is turned inside out. But in *C. pisiformis* even Leuckart found such forms with a normal head growing on a thin neck into the canal which he described as a scolex just starting to evaginate. In this he was wrong, because similar forms may be discovered in all cysticerci under certain circumstances without there being any connection with their evagination.

While studying old cysticerci from the brain, most of them being necrotic to some extent and at a stage of resorption, we discovered scolices of normal appearance as in the adult cestode growing on thin necks to varying distances into the entrance canal (Fig. 18) and, sometimes, protruding even onto the bladder surface (Fig. 19, Plate XI, Fig. 1 and 2). Conclusive proof of these forms of cysticerci can be obtained only by reconstruction. In overage and dead parasites these forms were relatively frequent not only in the brain, but even in the muscle tissue. In one of our observations, for example, this form was found in 8 out of 14 highly autolyzed parasites examined. The microscopical anatomy of the scolex and the neck was in relative accord with that of the adult cestode. Only in some instances the neck, mostly protruding from the wall at the outermost portion of the entrance canal, was much thin-

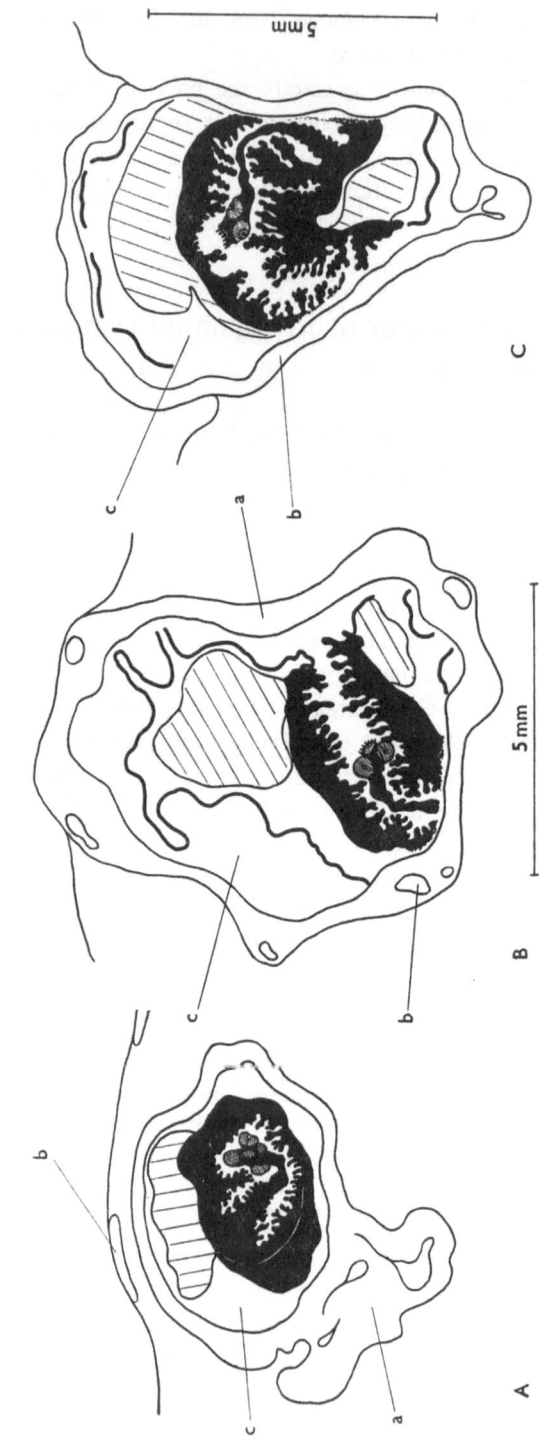

Fig. 18. A, B, C — Schematic reconstruction of the parenchymatous portion of partly resorbed cerebral cysticerci, in which an outgrown scolex on a neck was found. a — connective tissue encapsulation; b — vessels; c — exudate.

68

ner than under normal conditions. In one observation of a massive cysticercosis, in which the parasites were almost identical with the cysticerci of swine, this outgrown scolex was, in one instance, discovered still inside the originally coiled, invaginated canal with its characteristic, histological structure (Plate XXV, Fig. 3 and 4). The same findings were obtained even from histological studies of some dead *C. bovis* recovered from the musculature of cattle, but these cysticerci were shrivelled and de-

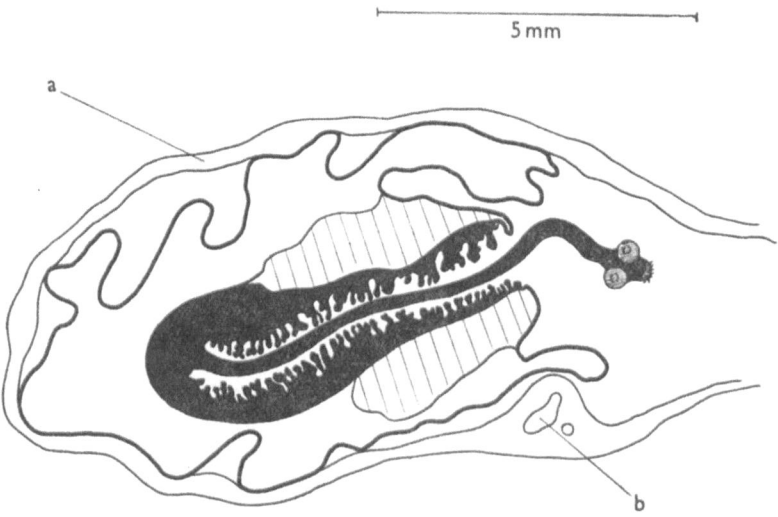

Fig. 19. Scheme of a longitudinal section through a shrivelled cerebral cysticercus with a scolex growing from the invaginated canal up to the opening on the bladder surface. a — connective tissue encapsulation; b — vessels. This is a reconstruction of the cysticercus, depicted in Plate XIX, Fig. 2 and in Plate XXVI, Fig. 2.

formed by the exudate and by autolytic processes. Therefore, attempts have been made to recover these forms from fresh material. We actually found some which, although dead, were not yet autolyzed and were thus able to discover in them the scolices growing to different distances into the spiral canal (Plate XI, Fig. 3 and 4). We even succeeded in discovering a form which was not only protruding from the opening of the bladder wall in a similar way to that observed in some cerebral forms of *C. cellulosae*, but in which the scolex on its thin neck reached the pointed pole of the bladder. Later, we found viable cysticerci with a scolex growing out of the bladder, their activity being similar to that of a cysticercus after evagination. Cysticerci with an outgrown scolex were found in the material of *C. pisiformis* and *C. crassiceps* (Plate XI, Fig. 5). Recently, a similar process was also observed in *Coenurus skrjabini* and in the larvae of *Multiceps endothoracicus*.

## 11. Differences between evagination and outgrowth of the scolex

It is relatively easy to evaginate mechanically a live cysticercus from its completely translucent bladder, but the bladder frequently becomes damaged. The first portion to turn into normal position during evagination is the invaginated surface

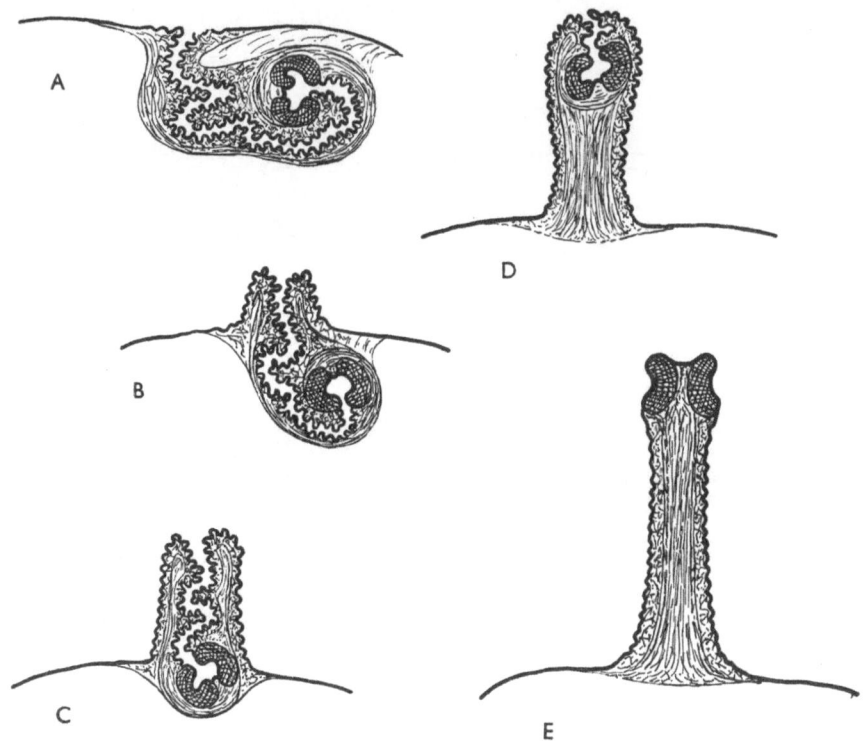

Fig. 20. Schematic illustration of the course of evagination in *C. bovis*.

of the spiral canal close under its opening on the bladder wall. The remaining portion reverses into normal position by gradually growing into an attenuated, obtuse cone with transverse rugae. Evagination becomes completed with the eversion of the suckers and the rostellum (Fig. 20). The suckers show signs of typical motion, this becoming usually arrested by fixation. The expanded position of the fixed suckers is characteristic making the peak of the scolex appear as if pressed in.

Up to the present, the process of spontaneous evagination of the cysticercus has been studied mainly from a physiological aspect. An initial period at a temperature of 38°C which activates the parasite is important for this process. This fact was pointed out by DE RYCKE and VAN GREMBERG (1965), who studied the evagination of scolices of *Echinococcus granulosus*. The fundamental importance of scolex evagination of the echinococcus to successful in vitro cultivation of the adult form was demonstrated by SMYTH (1967). CAMPBELL (1963) studied the effect of some surface-active agents after finding that evagination of the scolices could be stimulated by some standard household detergents (CAMPBELL and RICHARDSON 1960). He concluded that the evagination stimulus provided by bile salts can be attributed to their surface-active properties. DE RYCKE and VON GREMBERG (1966) observed in experiments with *Cysticercus pisiformis* that bile salt solutions are most effective at a concentration of 0·004M, the pH 4·5 being the approximate lower limit of their efficacy. In their opinion, no conclusive statement as to the role of surface tension in the evagination of the cysticercus can be made on the basis of present information. The course of evagination and the function of the individual tissues of the cysticercus in it will have to be studied with morphological experimental methods.

When evaginating a dead cysticercus, more pressure has to be applied and, often, the invaginated portion becomes damaged particularly if autolysis has started. In such instances the bladders are opaque or completely clouded and of brownish colour. The shape of the evaginated dead cysticercus is practically the same as that of the live cysticercus except that the former is longer, because the invaginated canal is longer in the older forms. When the scolex in the canal is outgrown it appears very suddenly during evagination, the moment of its appearance in the opening depending, naturally, on the length of the outgrowing neck. If the neck is long and has reached almost the opening of the canal the scolex appears as soon as pressure is applied to the invaginated portion, if it is short, the scolex appears later in the course of evagination. This evagination with the scolex coming out first always suggests an outgrown scolex because a normal scolex can appear only at the very end of evagination. The outgrown portion can be clearly demonstrated on an evaginated and dead cysticercus. The rostellum is elevated above the suckers, which are followed by an attenuated, often smooth neck. The outgrown portion is always less folded than the reversed surface of the spiral canal and the longer the outgrown portion, the smoother its surface. In the live outgrown forms, however, the scolex is the same as in the normally evaginated ones and the elevation of the rostellum in the outgrown dead scolices is a consequence of the loss of tonus in the musculature. Even spontaneous evagination can occur in cysticerci, which have remained in their intermediate hosts. In cysticerci of cattle we have often observed evaginated scolices, but this evagination was never complete, at least the rostellum and the suckers were still invaginated in the anterior end of the evaginated parasite. All these cysticerci were enclosed in necrotic exudate; the solid, evaginated portion recessing from the bladder wall could always be demonstrated, but not the invaginated canal. In older *C. cellulosae* it may sometimes be possible to discover the process of evagination in the intermediate host, since the tissue reaction and heavy exudation occur only after the death of the cysticercus; by contrast, in *C. bovis* the tissue reaction and exudation seem frequently to be responsible for the death of the parasite and its spontaneous evagination before its complete autolysis. In *C. cellulosae*, the process of evagination is even more complicated because it starts inside this outer covering (Plate XII, Fig. 2), whereby the typical sequence in the origin of the solid body and the evagination of the suckers and the rostellum at the end of this process are the same.

## 12. Origin and microscopical anatomy of the outgrown scolices

The morphology of the forms with an outgrown scolex indicates very clearly that this is not an evagination of the invaginated scolex of the cysticercus but the active growth of a thin neck bearing the scolex in its normal position on its top, proceeding from within the invaginated portion of the cysticercus. This state is in accord with the initial period of growth of the adult cestode after evagination and its attachment to the intestine of the definitive host preceding strobilation. Our findings suggest that in the cysticerci the cells of the zone of growth lying close beneath the suckers, start to proliferate at a certain period even if the parasite remains in the tissue of its intermediate host.

In the cysticerci, this zone of growth can be demonstrated very clearly and we detected it in all examined species and forms of cysticerci. It consists of cell elements packed closely under the cuticle of the last part of the invaginated canal close to its blind ending with the suckers and the rostellum (Plate XXV, Fig. 1). This density of cells in such a short section is responsible for an elongation of their nuclei into narrow, spindleshaped formations measuring 12—15 μm in length, their maximum width being 1—2·5 μm. Staining with Giemsa colours the membrane of the nucleus and the coarse particles of chromatin a brilliant blue; the corpuscles inside the nucleus resembling nucleoli colour violet. The strongly basophilic cytoplasm is linked to the elongated ends of the nuclei. This demonstrable elongation of the cells is particularly marked in *C. cellulosae* and in *C. bovis*. Also the height of the layer attaining approximately 15 μm, suggests a dense aggregation of cells in a very short distance arranged more or less in a single row. It contains three-times more cells than the remaining parts of the canal. In the transitional forms of cerebral cysticerci, these cells are even more remarkable for their basophilic plasma, their height attaining 8—10 μm, that of their ovoid nuclei 5 μm with a diameter of 3 μm. We often discovered smaller, highly basophilic cells, which were about 6 μm high and contained two nuclei. Even the overall height of the cell layer (approximately 18 μm) suggests cell multiplication, but the cells are no longer arranged in a single row. In the typical forms of old cerebral cysticerci the differentiation of the zone of growth is particularly distinct, the aggregation of cells being 4-times greater than that under the cuticle of the other portion of the spiral canal. However, the cells are so densely packed that their plasma seems to coalesce into a homogeneous rim. The size of the nuclei with the outstanding nucleoli is practically the same; the nuclei are ovoid, 6 μm long and

3·5—4·5 µm wide. The cells of the subcuticular layer are thus noticeably differentiated from the minute cells of the parenchyma with nuclei measuring 3·5—4 µm in length and 2·5 µm in width.

While studying the zone of growth of subcuticular cells after an artificial evagination of the cysticercus, we observed it to pass in a short distance close beneath the suckers into a loosely arranged row of less high subcuticular cells (Plate XXV, Fig. 2). The parenchyma of this section was almost completely lacking calcareous corpuscles. The longitudinal cords of the main muscle fibres separating the subcuticular layer from the mid-parenchyma of the body were more marked. The course of the lateral excretory canals was very twisted. Of a similar histological appearance was also the short neck with the scolex starting to arise from its peak in the outgrowing forms except that the conspicuous cells of the zone of growth were distributed along the whole length of the attenuated neck. Its central portion constisting of a thin parenchyma, passed uninterrupted into the compact fibrous tissue, which is typical of the body of the evaginated cysticercus. In forms in which the neck had reached the surface of the bladder, we found a marked, histological difference between the structure of this neck and that of the portion originating from the evagination of the invaginated canal. The axis of the evaginated portion consisted of compact, fibrous tissue; the subcuticular layer was packed with calcareous corpusles, the surface folded in deep, regular folds. The surface of the outgrown portion was less folded, the folds were not so deep and less regular. The subcuticular layer consisted of parenchyma with a system of fibres and canals branched towards the surface; calcareous corpuscles were very scarce in comparison with the evaginated portion. The more marked multiplication of subcuticular cells was restricted to the region close beneath the suckers. The central portion of the neck consisting of parenchymal tissue arranged in a network with few cells but a relatively large number of flame cells, was very conspicuous. When comparing the histological structure of the scolex and the outgrown neck of cysticerci with conditions in the scolex and the neck of adult cestodes in the intestine, we found a remarkable scarcity of cells in the tissues of the outgrown forms. In the cestode the subcuticular layer is high, consisting of several rows of elongated elements resembling those in the zone of growth of the cysticercus. The most striking feature of the cestode is the density of cells in the central portion between the longitudinal canals and the musculature, containing numerous small cells with dark nuclei. These are practically nonexistent in the outgrown forms. In the adult cestode they are believed to constitute the anlage of the reproductive organs differentiating during the gradual strobilation of the cestode body. Their absence in the outgrown forms of the cysticercus and the general histological appearance of these forms prove that this is only a protracted proliferation of the larvae and not the qualitatively different growth of the adult cestode.

While the proliferation of the bladder is a property of adaptation of the larval stage, ensuring its adjustment to various conditions of the external environment, the character of the zone of growth in the sucker region is very different in its nature.

From this cell anlage the whole postembryonic development of the invaginated portion of the cysticercus is started and consequently also the morphogenesis of the future cestode. Its proliferation in overage cysticerci (Fig. 21) leading to the outgrowth of the completely formed scolex into the invaginated canal indicates that the initial growth of the young cestode is, at first, not stimulated by environmental conditions in the intestine of the definitive host, but is a continuation of larval growth

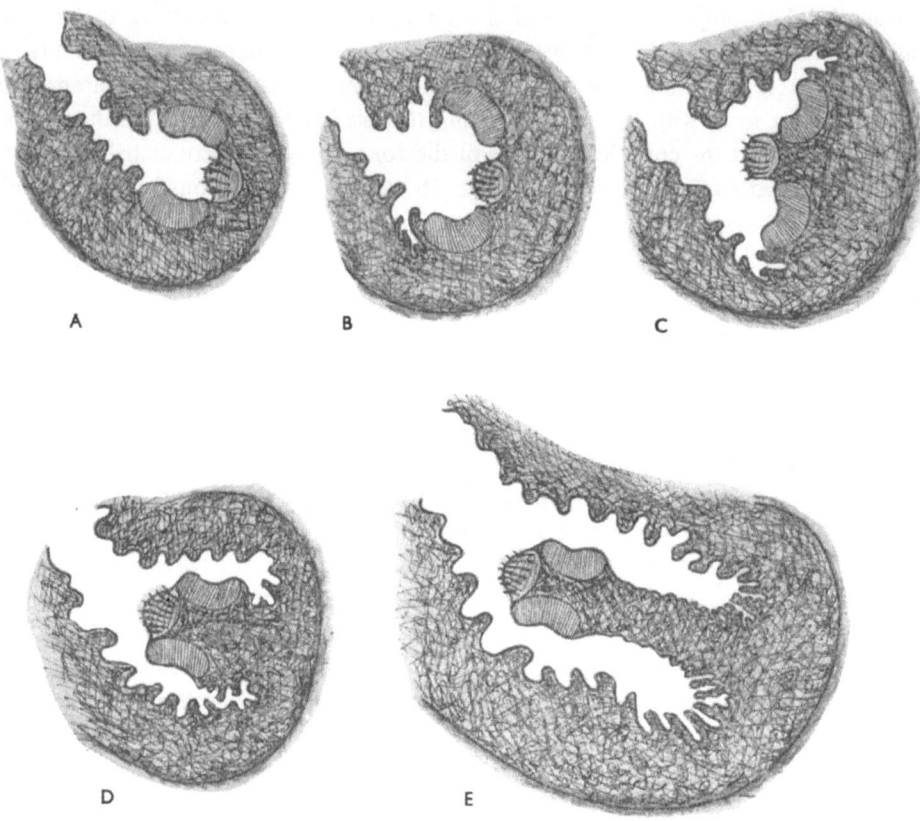

Fig. 21. Scheme illustrating the successive proliferation of the zone of growth in the region of the invaginated scolex (A, B, C) bringing the rostellum and suckers into normal position (D) and leading to the successive outgrowth of the scolex on its neck into the invaginated canal (E) in overage cysticerci.

setting in at a certain age of the larva. It seems only logical that such growth of a cysticercus, persisting and aging in its intermediate host, should become restricted to a mere proliferation and to the outgrowth of the neck without leading to any further development. These forms with an outgrown scolex are difficult to identify especially in cerebral cysticercosis, because only fragments of the cysticercus are found in an old and often calcified scar. Although this morphology of the parasite is visible in some photomicrographs in articles by BICKERSTAFF et al. 1956, PIAZZA and GADDO 1962, these writers failed to observe it and described it as an invaginated scolex. Neither MARCHAND (1879) nor MENNICKE (1897) found an explanation for similar findings, as pointed out in a previous paper (ŠLAIS 1960) in which also attention was given to these outgrown forms in *C. cellulosae* from the brain. No such forms have been recorded from *C. bovis*. They have been observed in *C. pisiformis* but not explained by some earlier investigators. In *C. crassiceps* which reproduces by budding and of which various forms at different developmental stages can be found in one host, such findings are not infrequent. However, these also are believed to be evaginated scolices as, for example, by FREEMAN (1962). Special forms discovered by the writer during the transplantation of cysticerci to another host, are a typical example of the continuing proliferation of the bladder and the scolex end in the larva. The various stages of spotaneous evagination in *C. bovis* were pictured in detail by DEWHIRST et al. (1963).

# 13. Importance of the bladder for the development of the cysticercus

As shown in the preceding chapters the bladder of the cysticercus constitutes a temporary organ which, in its morphology, depends on the mode of development and on the localization of the parasite in the intermediate host. The bladder ensures the existence of the larva in the organism and the tissues of the intermediate host and also its adaptation to abnormal conditions, for example in another intermediate host or organ not commonly involved in its life cycle (Fig. 22).

The mother bladder originates from the oncosphere after its localization in the intermediate host. It is covered with a cuticular layer of mucopolysaccharides lying on a network of muscle fibres which is placed on a layer of reticular nature. The differentiated wall of the body is formed by the reticular skeleton after the central bladder cavity has originated. These muscle and reticular fibres can be found even in necrotic larvae and their origin can be determined as described later. After the histological differentiation of the wall, the scolex originates from the cell anlage which has been retained at one of the poles. Following this stage, the scolex, and with it the future cestode, and the bladder — a temporary embryonic organ — develop in a specialized way. In *C. crassiceps* the cavity of the mother bladder is pushed back to such an extent that the bladder retreats to one end of the larva. A similar development was noted also in the bladder of *C. pisiformis* and *C. tenuicollis*, the only difference being the larger size of the bladder. This form with the bladder at one of the body and the parenchymatous portion with the invaginated scolex at the other end, is characteristic of all cysticerci developing in the body cavities or in subcutaneous pseudocysts of the intermediate host. *C. cellulosae* and *C. bovis*, which develop

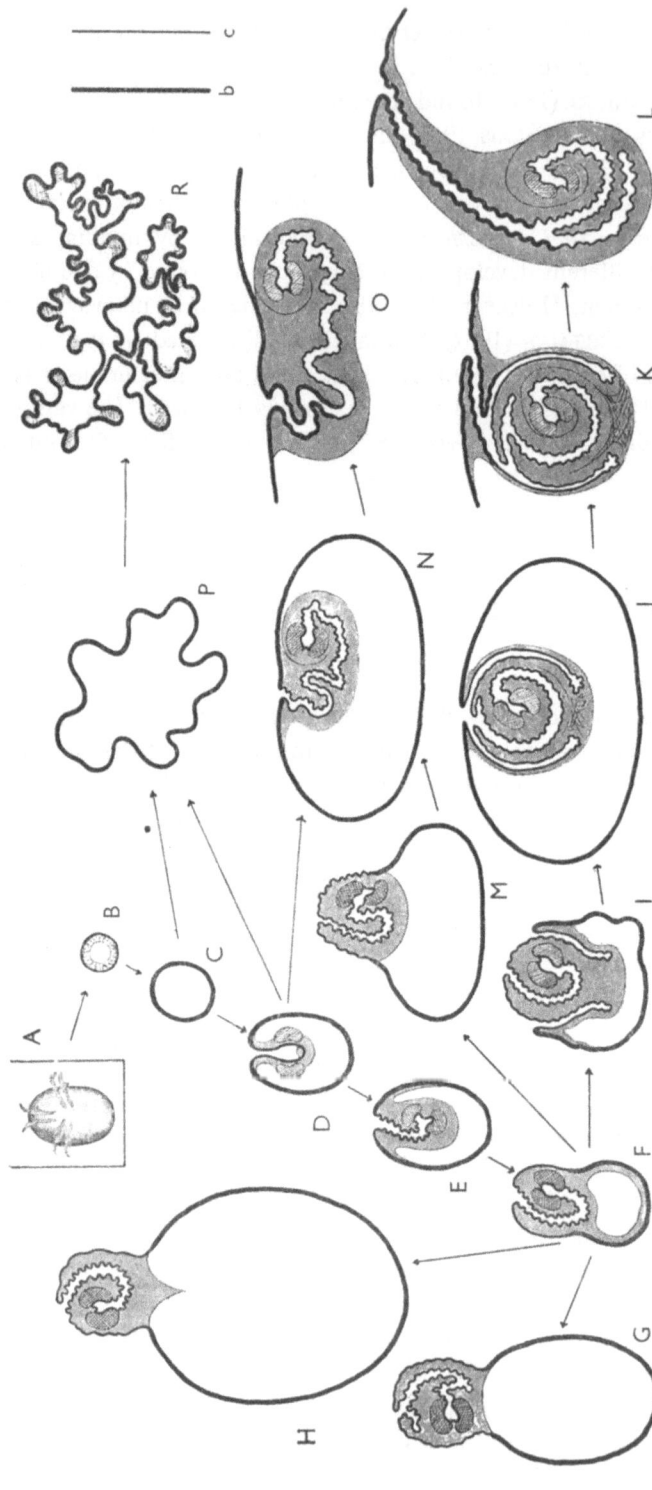

Fig. 22. Schematic illustration of the origin and differentiation of the cysticercus bladder as an adaptive larval organ. A — oncosphere after hatching; B — oncosphere changing into a mother bladder; C — mother bladder; D — mother bladder with developed scolex; E — continuing growth of spiral canal, F — development of the parenchymatous portion at the expense of the bladder; G — *C. pisiformis*; H — *C. tenuicollis*; I — proliferating bladder in the second developmental stage of *C. cellulosae*; J — typical *C. cellulosae*; K — transitional form of *C. cellulosae* with a developing entrance canal (only the parenchymatous portion has been drawn); L — typical parenchymatous portion of a *C. cellulosae* from the brain; M — proliferating bladder in the second developmental stage of *C. bovis*; N — typical *C. bovis*; O — parenchymatous portion of *C. bovis* with a developing entrance canal; P — proliferating bladder of a cysticercus; R — racemose form of cysticercus; b — bladder wall; c — surface of parenchymatous portion and of spiral canal.

76

directly in the tissues of the organs also pass through this stage during their early development; later, however, the growing bladder encloses completely in its cavity the parenchymatous portion with the scolex. Under different conditions, the bladder is most adaptable and can change both in size and form. An example of this is *C. cellulosae* in cerebral cysticercosis of man.

During the development of the scolex the cuticle invaginates into the cell anlage of the scolex and the organs of the scolex, suckers and the rostellum differentiate in the proliferating cell layer. The zone of growth in the region of the suckers continues in its proliferation and the spiral canal develops. Its length depends on the time for which the cysticercus remains in the intermediate host. All these forms are capable of invasion regardless of the length of the spiral canal. In the intestine of the definitive host, the cysticercus evaginates and becomes attached. The connecting part and the bladder are digested and the growth of the cestode starts from the zone of growth behind the suckers. At first this growth is a mere proliferation; after strobilation and the differentiation of the sexual organs the cysticercus begins to change into an adult cestode. The zone of growth initiating the growth of the neck is the primordial proliferation zone of the cells from which the scolex originated. This zone can already be found in the subcuticular layer of cells beneath the suckers in the invaginated cysticercus. In old cysticerci, which have persisted for a long time in their intermediate hosts, the proliferation of this zone was evidently started by old age. This process leads to the development of the invaginated cysticercus with the outgrown neck and scolex. We have found such living forms of *C. bovis* with normal sucker activity and it seems most probable that these forms can become attached to the intestine and be capable of further development.

The intra-uterine development of the mammalian embryo, especially the interstitial implantation of the embryo in the mucosa of the uterus, has often been classified as the period of parasitic relationship between the embryo and the mother. This specific kind of development influences some characteristic features of the mammalian embryo such as the early development of the trophoblast and the extra-embryonal mesenchyma, the development of the foetal envelopes and the placenta. The nutrition of the embryo, from the histiotrophic to the placental nutrition, reflects the complicated relationship between the embryo and the mother. The character of the nutrition, and equally, the complicated organization of the mammalian embryo and its embryonic organs cannot directly be compared with the conditions of parasites developing in the tissue. However, in consequence of the basically similar mode of living, there are some striking analogous features in the development and morphology of the transitional larval organs of a cysticercus and a mammalian embryo. The trophoblast of the mammalian embryo, ensuring conditions for the embedding and development of the embryo in the mucosa of the uterus, performs essentially the same function as the bladder of the cysticercus, which serves as mechanical protection and also functions in the metabolic contact of the larva with the surrounding tissue.

78

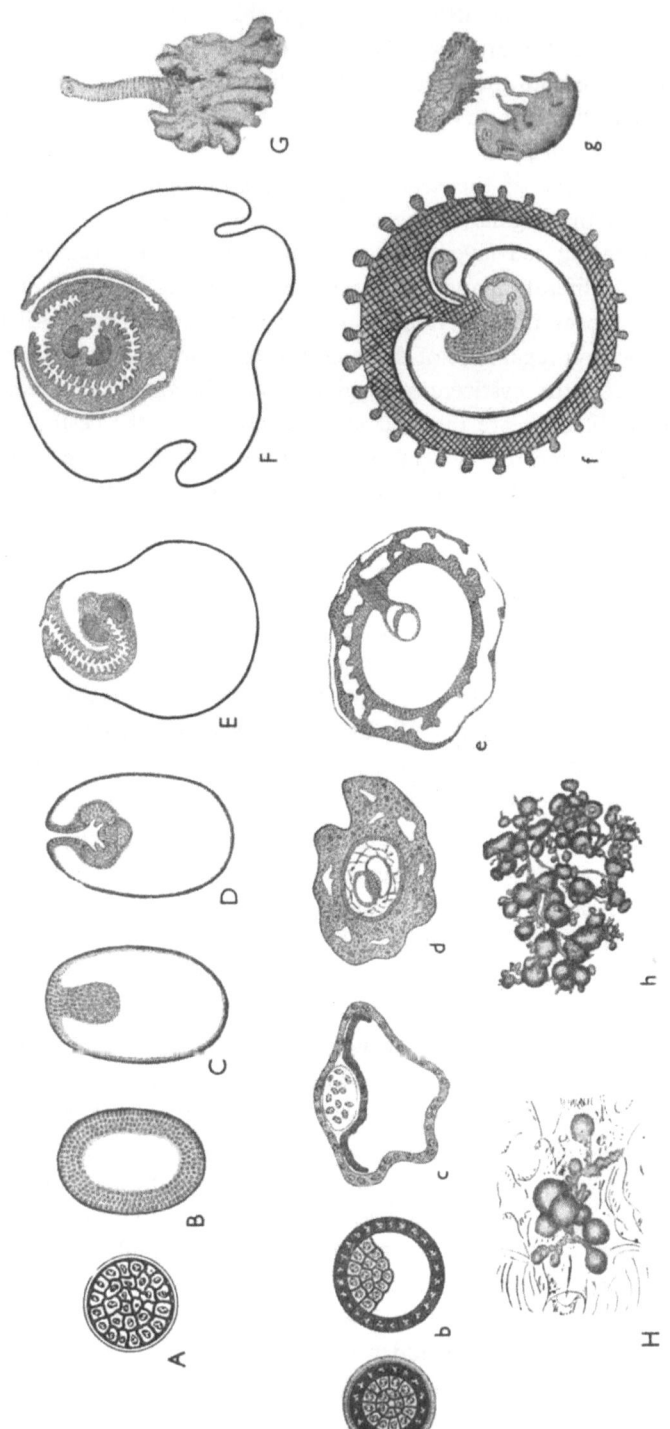

Fig. 23. Analogous features of the cysticercus bladder and the trophoblast of the mammalian embryo (scheme). A to F — development of the cysticercus; G — cysticercus after evagination of the scolex; a to f — development of the mammalian foetus and its envelopes; g — mammalian foetus with separated foetal envelopes joined to them by the umbilical cord after parturition; H — racemose cysticercus on the base of the brain; h — hydatid mole.

In the following text we have tried to point out all the characteristic stages of the development of the cysticercus bladder which resemble the development of the trophoblast and can be compared with it.

1) The first point of similarity is the early development of the bladder. In the cysticerci, the mother bladder with a differentiated wall originates first from the oncosphere. The proliferation of the cells continues only at one pole, forming a plug-like basis for the future development of the cestode (Fig. 23A—C). 2) Next the cuticle covering the bladder invaginates at the cell anlage and forms a canal. At the end of this canal the future organs of the scolex are becoming differentiated in a reversed position. The wall of the bladder develops as a larval organ and continues in this development, independently of the scolex. However, both these parts of the cysticercus must develop in mutual harmony to ensure the normal development of the larva; the same applies to the development of the trophoblast and the foetus (Fig. 23D). 3) In a later stage, the folded spiral canal connects the now differentiated scolex with the surface and the tissues of the bladder. The activities of growth are restricted to the terminal portion of the invaginated part round the suckers (Fig. 23E). 4) In the following developmental stage, the scolex of the cysticercus, enveloped in coverings which are most complicated in *C. cellulosae*, lies in the serous liquid of the bladder (Fig. 23F). 5) Finally, after the evagination of the cysticercus from the bladder in the intestine of the definitive host, the bladder and the spiral canal are digested and the cestode starts to grow from the scolex (Fig. 23G).

In the development of the trophoblast of the embryo attention may be drawn to the following features analogous to the development of the cysticercus bladder.

1) The first similarity is found in the very early development of the tropho-blast and the bladder. The blastocyst, a hollow ball, becomes differentiated from the morula of the mammalian embryo; the wall of the blastocyst formed by the epithe-lium of the trophoblast encloses the mass of germ cells at one pole (Fig. 23a—c). 2) The embryoblast then becomes differentiated into a germinal disk in which the blastodermic layers of the foetus originate. The development continues with the origin of the extra-embryonic mesenchyma. The histological development of the trophoblast terminates with the origin of the extra-embryonic coelom (Fig. 23d). 3) At a later stage the distinct separation of the embryo from the trophoblast, due to the origin of the umbilical stem, shows a close resemblance to the developmental situation in the cysticercus (Fig. 23e). 4) In its later development the foetus of the mammal is enclosed and protected, especially against mechanical blows, by the foetal envelopes (Fig. 23f). 5) After parturition, the placenta and the umbilical cord become separated (Fig. 23g).

Even under pathological conditions there is a great similarity in the properties of growth of the trophoblast and the bladder of the cysticercus. In some instances changes occur in the trophoblast which are believed to be caused by the early death of the embryo or, on the contrary, the embryo dies in consequence of these changes. The true cause has not yet been proved. The stroma of the chorionic villi succumbs to a hydropic degeneration and the epithelium proliferates distinctly. The villi change to cysts of various size resembling a grape-like formation; thus the hydatid mole originates (Fig. 23h). The bladder of the cysticercus, when localized in the brain of man, forms also occasionally large grape-like formations mainly at the base of the brain known as *Cysticercus racemosus* as described above (Fig. 23H). The individual groups of bladders originating from an autonomous proliferation of all components of the bladder wall are usually connected by pedunculate stalks. Nothing is known about the origin of this form and investigations are difficult because the scolex of the parasite, often still dystrophic, has been found in only a few instances. Mostly the scolex is not developed and only the bladder is proliferating excessively. In one observation the budding of the bladder wall and the origin of the typical grape-like formation was seen.

The congruent features demonstrated indicate the great morphogenetic influence of the milieu which causes the development of convergent adaptive organs in organisms as different as the embryo of mammals and the larva of cestodes.

# Localization of *Cysticercus cellulosae* and *Cysticercus bovis* in the organs

All papers dealing with the localization of the parasites in muscle cysticercosis have described only their development in the connective tissue which separates the finer and coarser bundles of muscle fibres (perimysium internum). These descriptions evidently presuppose the presence of the parasites in the connective tissue itself, in which also the inflammatory process develops and which, later, obliterates the original histological arrangement of the tissue surrounding the cysticerci (Plate XV, Fig. 1 and 2).

During our studies of young developmental stages of *C. cellulosae* from a massive cysticercosis in the musculature of swine we observed the larvae growing in the space lined with a single layer of endothelial cells (Plate XII, Fig. 1). This lining, sometimes resting only on a minimal layer of connective tissue, was found to adjoin the bundles of muscle fibres or the lobules of adipose tissue. In some places, however, this connective tissue layer was more prominent and contained more cells than usual. Gradually, the growing larvae dilated these spaces and their presence could be clearly demonstrated. Places containing more connective tissue were less dilated than the other parts of the wall surrounding these sites, which remained submerged in the growing bladder like a connective tissue septum (Plate XIV). In some instances, especially at the sites where the concentration of parasites was higher, the dilated places were filled with a precipitated, proteinic substance without cell elements which, in some places, was in direct contact with the parasite.

The histological character of the described spaces was typical of the lymphatic capillaries. There is little information available on the existence of lymphatic capillaries in the skeletal musculature. The few data found on this subject in the literature are contradictory and the only confirmed fact seeems to be the absence of lymphatic capillaries in the connective tissue enveloping the primary muscle fibres, i.e. in the endomysium, in contrast to the blood capillaries. In photomicrographs in the article by KOZMA and GELLER (1953) the lymphatic capillaries could be viewed clearly in the perimysium internum of the skeletal musculature. Their wall, in some places adjoining the muscle bundles, became dilated after the ligation of the main lymphatic vessels. A typical feature of the wall of the lymphatic capillaries is its solely endothelial make-up, the endothelial cells being larger than these in the blood capillaries. Thereby, the wall of the lymphatic capillary is indistinguishable from the surrounding connective tissue (ZHDANOV 1952) and no valves are present in its lumen, this being a feature differentiating the lymphatic capillary from the smallest lymphatic vessel. Often, the lymphatic capillaries have a much wider lumen than these vessels, however, this is often irregular, lacunary. Numerous small elevation are frequently found in its wall, coursing in circles on its periphery and functioning partly like valves. These were first observed by RECKLINGHAUSEN (1871) who stated that "the wall of the lymphatic capillary right down to its finest branches is provided with varicose elevations. These are often found at the crossing points of the network and appear so suddenly that transverse elevations protrude into the lumen. Thereby they are orientated in such a way that they function, to some extent, like valves".

There is no doubt that the concentration of connective tissue at the crossing points of the capillary network is particularly striking in the lymphatic capillaries of the skeletal musculature of swine. As mentioned in the foregoing text it resembles septa cutting into the distending bladder.

During the preparation of C. bovis recovered from the skeletal musculature of bovine animals, we observed these cysticerci to occur always in the thicker septum of connective tissue dividing the increased number of primary bundles of muscle fibres and never between these bundles (Plate XXIV, Fig. 3 and 4). These connective tissue septa formed by the crossing layers of fibrous connective tissue and communicating connective tissue bands, extend from them to the surface of the neighbouring bundles of muscle tissue (BENNINGHOF 1944). These membranes are interspersed with vessels and nerves and apparently also with the finest branches of the lymphatic network in which the cysticerci develop. Because the musculature of cattle contains considerably less adipose tissue than that of swine, the wall of these lymphatic interstices usually lies very close to the muscle bundles and is very difficult to observe. However, in serial section, the transition from the cavity into these lymphatic capillaries could be demonstrated even at a stage of advanced inflammatory encapsulation of the parasite. Since the connective tissue in the skeletal musculature of cattle is not reinforced at the crossing points of the lymphatic capillary network, no connective tissue septum was found to cut into the bladders of C. bovis. Cysticerci situated in the dilated lymphatic spaces (up to the time of the more distinct development of the inflammation) are surrounded only by the connective tissue of these membranes which, in earlier accounts, was erroneously described as a fibrous encapsulation.

In cysticercosis of the heart we found parasites in these lymphatic spaces not only in the myocardium, but very often in the endocardium and epicardium. According to ZHDANOV (1952) the subendocardiac network of the lymphatic capillaries situated in the connective tissue of the endocardium, is most irregular and its loops are especially elongated in the papillary muscles. Short capillaries of the endocardiac network fuse with the intramyocardiac network, its capillaries being three-times larger in diameter than the blood capillaries. Because no larger lymphatic drainage vessels are present in the myocardium, the lymphatic capillaries of the myocardium mostly open directly into the lymphatic capillary network of the epicardium. The subepicardiac lymphatic network is well developed and drains the lymph of the endo-cardium and of the wall of the heart.

The connective tissue of the myocardium being, in fact, more marked than that of the skeletal musculature, communicates with the connective tissue of the epicardium and endocardium. FEDYAY (1961) demonstrated lymphatic capillaries in the connective tissue between the primary bundles and the groups of bundles of the cardiac muscle, in the coarser connective tissue septa and around the adventitia of the vessels. Therefore, the lymphatic capillaries in the myocardium always proceed through sites with more connective tissue. However, in the thick connective tissue layer of the epicardium the lymphatic capillaries are more numerous and the network less regular.

Particularly noteworthy is the localization of the parasites under the endo-cardium, namely on the papillary muscles, where often relatively large cysticerci were seen to bulge into the ventricle at the points of attachment of the chordae tendinae. According to DOBROVOLSKAYA-ZAYTSEVA (1961), the network of lymphatic capillaries is placed in the deep, collagenous, elastic layer of the endocardium, com-municating in some parts with the myocardium. The longest capillaries always ac-company the bundles of collagenous and elastic fibres of the endocardium and the mechanical properties of the thin layer of endocardiac connective tissue ensure the marked bulging of the parasites on the endocardiac surface without letting them break through into the cardiac cavities.

The proof of the localization of the cysticerci in the lymphatic capillaries in muscle cysticercosis brings up the question of the routes along which the young larvae move to these sites. The active penetration of the oncosphere through the intestinal wall and into the blood capillaries is a well-known fact as is their trans-portation by the bloodstream to the affected organs. In muscle cysticercosis it has to be supposed that the young larvae, while actively leaving the blood capillaries at the junction of the arterial and venous part, damage the walls. This hypothesis may be supported by the minute haemorrhagies observed in experimental studies of the early phases of cysticercosis development, which have also been mentioned in the older literature and emphasized by von MEYENBURG (1929). We were able to demonstrate hemosiderin in a minute focus in the connective tissue next to the wall of encapsulation of a cysticercus in the musculature of a bovine animal. This indicates that the oncospheres penetrate actively the lymphatic capillaries of the muscle, in which they develop, being bathed by the lymph. Thus, they are in direct metabolic contact with the lymph and their metabolic products are distributed throughout the whole organism by the outflowing lymph, reaching the blood far quicker than when growing directly in the connective tissue as has been believed up till the present.

In a multiple cerebral cysticercosis the pia mater is the most affected site. Ac-cording to the reports of surveys by various authors on the localization of the cerebral cysticercus, 2/3rd to 3/4th of cerebral cysticerci were found in the pia mater, 1/4th in the cerebral ventricles and only 1/6th—1/8th in the deeper layers of the white matter and the gray matter of the cerebrum. This is in keeping with our findings except for one case of an extremely massive cysticercosis of the brain, in which parasites were found to be distributed over the whole organ. A certain uniformity of localization cannot be confirmed only on the grounds of discovering solitary parasites in the brain. In an excessive cerebral cysticercoss, there is a marked correspondence

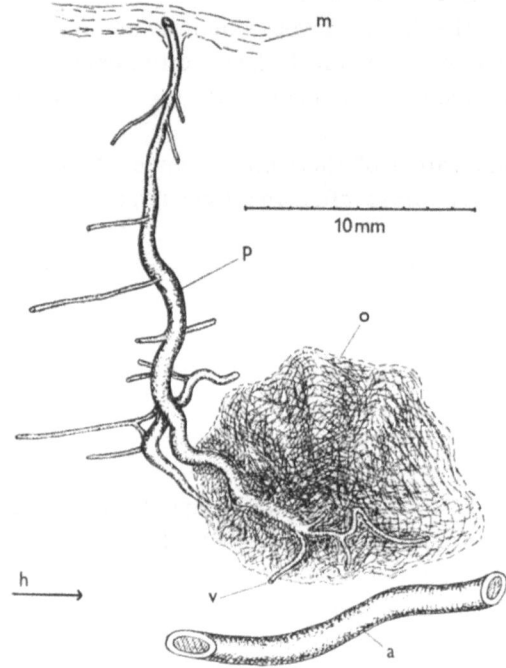

10 mm

Fig. 24. Reconstruction of the precapillary in the brain cortex showing its relationship to the connective tissue encapsulation of the cysticercus. The vessel in front of the lesion is dilated and filled with precipitate. Its branches continuing past the connective tissue encapsulation are of normal appearance. m — surface of the brain cortex, p — precapillary, v — branches of the precapillary beyond the site where it grows into the connective tissue encapsulation of the parasite, o — only part of the encapsulation was drawn, h — border between the gray and white matter in the brain cortex; a — section of the artery at this site.

between the localization of the parasites in the brain tissue and the course of its vessels. In these instances it is evident that the oncospheres become lodged in the terminal capillaries of the cortex and the central gray matter. There, the parasites carried to these sites continue to develop, because their localization offers no other possibility. In one observation we discovered in a series of slides of a parasite, recovered from the cortex at the border of the white and gray matter, the termination of a dilated precapillary with a thrombosis of its lumen and of all branches situated closer to the surface of the brain in the encapsulating connective tissue of the parasite. In this case, the generally spherical parasitic cyst was digitally extended towards this vessel and the inflammatory process had spread also to its wall (Fig. 24).

In cysticercosis of the pia mater, however, the larvae seem to migrate actively from the vessels to the cavum leptomeningicum where conditions, being similar to those in the lymphatic capillaries, are suitable for their development. According to the exhaustive study by KLIKA (1959), the endothelial-like lining of the subarachnoid cavity is absolutely uninterrupted and the larvae dilate it while growing. They prefer naturally to grow in the more spacious portions of the cavum leptomeningicum, i.e. the cerebral grooves and especially, the cisternae. This explains the remarkably frequent occurrence of the parasite in the fissura lateralis cerebri. Also we found completely developed parasites lying freely in the cisterna valleculae lat. cerebri and in the cisterna v. cerebralis magnae between the pons and the girus hippocampi. When growing in the less spacious parts of the subarachnoid cavity, the meshes of its network cut into the enlarging bladder like septa especially at the sites where they accompany the bridging vessels. We observed this to occur mainly in cysticerci localized in the low subarachnoid cavity of the cerebellum.

No answer has been found yet to the problem about the routes, along which these free cysticerci move to the cerebro-spinal fluid of the ventricles, in which they attain the largest size. In our observation of a massive cerebral cysticercosis we found parasitic cysts close under the lining of the ventricles, bulging into its cavity like peas. The vessels were dilated and the subependymal layer was greatly attenuated. In two instances the wall was broken and the scolex portion of the parasite protruded into the ventricle like a polypous formation, while its bladder was still occupying the subependymal cavity (Fig. 8). Nearby, we found several scarred, subependymal, fibrous capsules without parasites (Plate XXVI, Fig. 3). These findings suggest that, sometimes, the parasite growing under the subependymal layer breaks through the bulging wall and falls into the cerebrospinal fluid (CSF). In two instances the parasite became trapped in the broken wall and continued its development there. This may suggest one of the routes along which the cysticerci move to the ventricles and develop into freely swimming bladders in the CSF contrary to the generally accepted belief that the oncospheres move directly into the CSF. Our findings show that subependymally localized, developing cysticerci are passively liberated into the CSF and do not move actively into it, while from there they may be transported by the flow of the CSF into the fourth ventricle, this being the site where most of these free cysticerci were observed to cause noteworthy symptoms (KAHLDEN 1897, SCHÖPPLER 1906, HERZOG 1913, HENNER and JEDLIČKA 1920 a.o.). Should the larva by then attain a larger size it may get caught in the third ventricle where it usually blocks the aqueduct (KRATTER and BÖHMIG 1897, DVOŘÁČEK 1949 a.o.). HEILMAN (1932) discovered a cysticercus even in the foramen of Monro.

Interesting also is the abnormal localization of *C. cellulosae* in an infection of man. In swine this cysticercus is found mostly in the abdominal muscles, the diaphragm, the tongue, the heart, the masseters, the intercostal muscles, the pectoral and cervical muscles and in some muscles of the posterior extremities. In a massive infection OSTERTAG (1913) found parasites in the nodes, the subcutaneous fat and in the brain, while in an even more extensive infection parasites were present also in the liver and the lungs. The frequent finding of these parasites in the brain and the eyes of man are by some investigators believed to be misleading evidence because of the relatively easy discovery of the cysticerci in these organs. However, the predeliction of the parasites for the central nervous system (CNS) even in a generalized infection was confirmed by DIXON and LIPSCOMBS (1961), who examined and observed for a long time 450 soldiers of the British Army in India, all infected with cysticercosis.

Interesting results were obtained by MAZZOTTI et al. (1965) in studies of spontaneous and experimental *C. cellulosae* infection in abnormal hosts. Five of the 270 dogs examined were positive. Of these, cysticerci in the brain were discovered in four, and a generalized cysticercosis in one dog. In an experimental infection the parasites were localized mainly in the brain. In a solitary finding of the parasite in a cat and also after the experimental infection of this animal, the parasites were found mainly in the brain. Experimental infection of a spider monkey (*Ateles geoffroyi*) and a coati (*Nasua narica*) resulted always in the infection of the brain; in some of the experimental animals cysticerci were also present in the muscles, the heart, the liver and the lung. Experimental infections of rats and mice were unsuccessful, only in a single, spontaneously infected rat (out of a total of 316 examined animals) was *C. cellulosae* found in the brain.

On the basis of reports from the literature and also of our own observations concerned with the exclusive localization of the parasites in the region of the branches of the a. carotis externa in a multiple cysticercosis of the meninges and the brain we came to the conclusion that the course of embolisation of the larvae entering the bloodstream was responsible for this localization. This depends, naturally, on the laws governing the bloodstream and on the anatomy of the main arterial trunks of the attacked intermediate host, as was pointed out by SCHWARZHAUT (1929). Only after becoming arrested in the capillary bed do the larvae start to move actively to the sites of their definitive location in the organs. The embolisation of the oncospheres of *T. solium* mainly in the large arteries receding from the arcus aortae, has been confirmed also by demonstrations of muscular and subcutaneous cysticercosis, occurring mostly in the upper parts of the trunk, the upper extremities and in the neck and the head. Also in support of this are our findings of cysticerci in a muscle cysticercosis located mainly in the pectoral and brachial muscles.

The restriction of *C. bovis* mostly to the masseters and the heart of bovine animals seems to depend also on anatomical conditions of the circulatory system. This has been confirmed in France by CHABASSE and GENTHON (1962), who found cysticerci in these sites in 83% of all animals examined. Other sites of localization of the cysticerci in cows are the cervicle muscles, the diaphragm, the pectoral and the intercostal muscles. Solitary parasites may be found also in other organs. This, however, occurs mostly if the incidence is high, but very seldom if incidence is low. Sometimes, particularly in cattle, a *C. bovis*-like cysticercus was found mainly in the liver. This cysticercus has been recorded repeatedly from the giraffe and PRICE (1961) even succeeded in infecting man with it. The eggs obtained from this experimental infection were fed to calves and caused a generalized cysticercosis with the highest incidence in the liver. In view of slight divergencies in the structure of the mature proglottids of the adult form the author described it as a new variety under the name *Taenia saginata* var. *giraffae*.

The undetectable presence of *C. bovis* in only lightly infected cattle is still one of the main sources of human infection with adult cestodes even under the most advanced hygienic conditions and mandatory inspection of the carcasses at the abattoir (DESPRÉS and RAUSCH 1961).

# Cysticercosis of livestock and man

## 1. Introduction

Muscle cysticercosis of livestock not only greatly reduces the profits yielded by these animals, but constitutes also a dangerous source of infection to man with the adult cestode. The consumption of underdone meat in addition to the infection of persons handling raw meat, is the most common source of infection of man with either *Taenia solium* or *Taeniarhynchus saginatus*. The exclusive predeliction of the adult forms of both these cestodes for man suggests their relatively recent phylogenetical adaptation. Since the scolex of *T. solium* is armed with hooks and that of *Trh. saginatus* is not, they can easily be identified by their scolices. Less simple is their identification on the grounds of the morphology of the mature proglottids. A recent study by VERSTER (1967) showed that the most important diagnostic sign is the vaginal sphincter, which is present in *Trh. saginatus* and absent in *T. solium*. The number of uterine branches in the gravid segment is most variable and, in Verster's opinion, not a suitable character for distinguishing these two species. She also maintained that *T. solium* is less rare than generally believed, because its apparant scarcity is often due to errors in identification. In our opinion this may applies mainly to conditions in South Africa, but not to Europe, where *T. solium* has become almost extinct. The disappearance of this cestode and the increased frequency of *Trh. saginatus* was noted by OSTERTAG (1895). The situation in Czechoslovakia was reviewed by PETRŮ and VOJTĚCHOVSKÁ (1963). From a group of 581 cestode-infested persons from Prague and surroundings, these authors recovered only *Trh. saginatus*. The records of PAWLOWSKI (1964) from the Poznan district, covering the years 1953—1964, list only 8 cases of *T. solium* infection against 1,200 cases of *Trh. saginatus* infection.

Of utmost importance in the epidemiology of taeniases are the intermediate hosts. For *T. solium* these are mainly the domestic pig or the wild hog. The occurrence of *C. cellulosae* in other intermediate hosts, where it may be most numerous, is not restricted to the muscles, for it may selectively parasitize the CNS. The list of other intermediate hosts includes sheep, red deer, fallow deer, gazelle, dog, cat, bear, monkey and also man. HEINZ and ARON (1966) maintained that the cysticerci in abnormal hosts (cat, dog, baboon and man) which were identified as *C. cellulosae* showed features different from those of *C. cellulosae* in the pig. They also suggested that the number and size of hooks from cysticerci of the pig indicated the presence of two different populations of cysticerci. In connection with the specific relationship of *T. solium* to man there is the interesting finding of *C. cellulosae* in the brain of a White hand gibbon (*Hylobates lar lar*) which, being recovered from the brain and fed to a young male of this same ape species, developed into a mature cestode (CADIGAN et al. 1967). This demonstrates that not only man but also the ape can be both the intermediate and the definitive host of this cestode.

Very different is the relationship between man and *Trh. saginatus*, the cysticercus of which has never been found in man. The few recorded findings are generally regarded as being completely unconvincing. The absence of *C. bovis* in man cannot be explained by the inability of the oncosphere to emerge from the egg of *Trh. saginatus* during its passage through the gut. The results of experiments by GÖNNERT et al. (1967) support the hypothesis that eggs of *T. solium* must pass through the stomach before the embryophores disintergrate easily in the small intestine and thus produce a successful infection. Comparative tests with eggs of *Trh. saginatus* gave similar results. The range of intermediate hosts of *C. bovis* is very limited comprising only bovine animals. The complete disappearance of *T. solium* and the predominant frequency of *Trh. saginatus* in man in Europe is responsible for the distribution of cysticercosis on this Continent. In Czechoslovakia, for example, cysticercosis of swine is very rare and found only in imported animals. By contrast the incidence of cysticercosis of cattle is increasing and becoming a grave veterinary and health problem. The changed ratio in the frequency of these species seems to be related to changes in the breeding of swine and cattle (see p. 13).

## 2. Distribution of *C. cellulosae* in swine and man throughout the world

Attention has been given to this cysticercus mainly because man may become infected. There is no clear evidence available yet on the routes of this infection as is shown in the article by WEBBE (1967) on internal autoinfection. The fact that man can be a carrier of only *C. cellulosae* was demonstrated in Europe after the introduction of mandatory inspection of the carcasses at the abattoirs and the gradual improvement of hygienic conditions in swine breeding. Cysticercosis of man affecting mainly the CNS and the eye, this being a characteristic site and not only a means of easy diagnosis, as was originally believed, provides a good indication of infection because of the severity of the clinical manifestation. In Germany in the 60s of the last century, Virchow recorded at post mortem about 2% of cysticercosis; in 1882 the records of the hospital Charité in Berlin show cysticercosis in 0·26% of all post mortem examinations, but only 0·16% in 1903. The records of the ophthalmic clinics show a similarly rapid decrease in the frequency of the cysticercus. This fact correlates with the records of the Berlin abattoirs in the year in which mandatory meat inspection was introduced: in 1883, the incidence of cysticercosis in swine was 0·6%, in 1902 only 0·03%. Except for the years following close after the First World War, this decrease continued and, at present, cysticercosis of swine is almost nonexistant in Central Europe. Also cysticercosis of man is very rare (ŠLAIS 1965). More frequent is the incidence of cysticercosis in the East-European countries. In Poland STEPIEN (1962) recorded 132 cases identified over the years 1936—1961 and stated that the incidence of cerebral cysticercosis in all patients admitted to the neurological clinics was 0·29%. BOJARSKI and WALESZKOWSKI (1963) described 16 instances of cerebral cysticercosis from Lodź found in the years 1948—1962. As a result, cerebral cysticercosis was subjected to experimental research (KEPSKI et al. 1963). The recent finding (PRZEORSKA 1967) of C. cellulosae in the eye of a 10-year old boy underlines the present importance of the problem in Poland. A similar frequency of cysticercosis has also been recorded from the Balkans; from Yugoslavia (Bosnia) by FERKOVICH (1964), from Roumania by MÉRA et al. (1961), from Bulgaria by GANCHEV (1961), the latter describing the treatment of this infection. Also here, AVLAVIDOV and KOVKHAZOV (1965) discovered during their studies of the cestodes of man T. solium only 6 times, but Trh. saginatus 216 times. All these writers drew attention to the remarkable decrease of cysticercosis in swine during this period (0·001%). Conditions are similar in the U.S.S.R., especially in its European part. Solitary cases are still on record (ANTONOV 1966; SAMSONOV and MESHKOVA 1967 describe a case of autoinfection). SALGANIK (1967) in his monograph dealing with clinical observations described 81 cases of cerebral cysticercosis treated in Moldavia within the last 20 years. In western and southern Europe, an increased incidence of cysticercosis has been recorded only from Spain, while in Italy this infection was almost unknown. Only recently solitary cases were recorded by PIAZZA and GADDO (1962), d'ANDREA et al. (1964). In France, the finding of only 3 cases of cysticercosis was made the subject of a communication (LAFON et al. 1957). Similarly in Portugal, only two cases have been reported (D'OLIVEIRA 1967).

Cysticercosis has often been more frequent among the soldiers of the colonial armies. An exhaustive analysis of 450 cases of cysticercosis among the soldiers of the British Army in India was presented by DIXON and LIPSCOMB (1961) demonstrating the frequent incidence of the infection in this country. New cases are still being recorded from India (SHOWRAMMA and REDY 1963) and also from Southeastern Asia and China, which is believed to be the classical region for the occurrence of cysticercosis (CHUNG and LEE 1935). This disease is also distributed all over Mongolia and Korea, while in Japan it is very rare and the few cases recorded may be infections acquired abroad (KITAOKA 1962). In Mohammedan countries, where pork consumption is forbidden by religion, cysticercosis of man is unknown. In the countries of the Near- and Middle-East, taeniases of man are frequent; in Syria Trh. saginatus was found in 2% of all patients with parasitic infection (DACCAK 1962) and also the incidence of cysticercosis in cattle is high. Cysticercosis of man has not been recorded. In Iran, the first case was described by AFSHAR (1967) who, therefore, revised all findings of cysticercosis of swine. Cysticercosis was found in 0·02 to 0·03% of 24,000 domestic pigs examined compared with 4% found in 4,800 wild hog. The author concludes that in Iran, where the Christian population consumes hog meat, the incidence of *T. solium* should be more frequent. Cysticercosis is not known in the Mohammedan countries of North and Central Africa, but is found in South Africa, where LIPSCHITZ et al. (1967) found cerebral cysticercosis even in small children. In Ghana, two cases have been recently recorded by ODAMTTEN and LAING (1967). In the years 1955—1965 GOLDSMITH (1966) found at autopsy 60 cases of cysticercosis in Africans of Rhodesia and Nyasaland. Serological cysticercosis tests were positive in 8·5% of Bantu. HEINZ and KLINWORTH (1965) considered cysticercosis to be the main cause of epilepsy among African patients of whom 12·7% reacted positively in serological tests. By contrast only 2% of epileptic Europeans were positive. PROCTOR et al. (1966) obtained sera for their investigation into serological diagnosis of cysticercosis from 48 Africans, in whom disease was confirmed. POWELL et al. (1966) described neurological complications in these patients. ELDON - DEW (1967) found by serological tests not only a high proportion of positive reactors in Natal, but also a close association with epilepsy and other nervous disorders in the African. In South Africa, however, cerebral coenurosis of man and its relationship to the racemose form of cysticercosis is still an unsolved problem. While in the U.S.A. cerebral cysticercosis is very rare and, according to TOMIYASU et al. (1966), only 30 cases have been reported in the literature, Mexico is the country with the highest incidence. BRICENO et al. (1961) alleged that cysticercosis was identified in 2·8—3·5% of all post mortem examinations. IZQUIERDO (1960) mentioned cysticercosis in 3·6% of autopsy records and in 11% of patients hospitalized at the neurological clinic in Mexico City. The reason for this is the high incidence of cysticercosis in swine and evidently also conditions under which pigs are bred. Great efforts are being made, therefore, to detect cysticerci at the abattoir (MAZZOTTI 1966) and to find effective measures for their elimination (BIAGGI et al. 1963, 1965, 1966). The authors recommend refrigeration at —20 °C for not less than 12 hours as the most effective method for destroying the parasites. This method does not affect the characteristics of the meat and is now generally used at abattoirs also against cysticercosis of cattle.

A similar incidence of infection is found also in Central and South America. In Guatemala, parasitological examinations performed in the years 1951—1960 revealed an incidence of 1·13% of *T. solium* and of 1·72% of *Trh. saginatus*; cysticercosis was diagnosed in 118 patients. In Central America and Panama, cysticercosis of swine was found to average 2·13% (ACHA and AGUILAR 1964). The first two autochthonous cases of cerebral cysticercosis in Cuba were described by MARIN et al. (1967). In Columbia, LOPEZ and ESCANDON (1964) recorded at autopsy an incidence of 0·7% over a period of 20 years. In Chile, cysticercosis was identified even more recently in 25 out of 202 patients examined for cerebral tumors (VARLETA et al. 1964). In Peru, cysticercosis has been studied for many years by Trelles, who based his research work on an analysis of 33 cases (ex. TRELLES 1961). Also in Brazil, great attention has been given to research on cysticercosis. SPINA - FRANCA (1956) recorded 50 cases of cerebral cysticercosis. The frequency of cysticercosis in the neurological clinic at Sao Paulo was 2·98% on average in the years 1947—1955. There are some records of cysticercosis from all other countries of Latin America, recently from Ecuador (GUERRERO 1965). Because this infection constitutes a grave health problem, systematic research is being performed in addition to case reports in order to develop convenient diagnostic methods (SPINA - FRANCA and CANELA in the years 1960—1964) and also therapeutic methods, treatment being mainly of a surgical nature (e.g. BULNES 1960, SAPUNAR and MORALES 1963).

## 3.   Histological evidence of cysticerci and their remnants in the tissues

A live cysticercus can be easily identified by the histological structure of its parasitic bladder or even of its fragments. A more difficult situation arises with very old and, therefore, degenerating parasites with tissues succumbing to regressive changes. This situation is very frequent in cysticercosis of man particularly in a not extensive infection or in one which has not affected important centres. After the death of the parasite and its autolysis the tissues of the host start to react to the products of autolysis thus greatly impeding the identification of the parasite's remnants. The first signs of degenerative changes are a stagnation of metabolic processes. The lacunae of the excretory system of canals in the parenchyma become dilated and filled with an at first amorphous, later coarsely granular substance which, sometimes, particularly in the bladder wall, resembles a pigment (Plate XVI, Fig. 5). These substances are of a natural, yellowish colour; the small granules stain blue with Giemsa, green with Goldner, the larger granules stain violet with Giemsa, red with Goldner and are PAS-positive. The surface layer of the parenchyma on the invaginated portion of the parasite is mostly largely permeated with these precipitates. After fixation we found in the uncollapsed bladder a minimum of precipitate, this being by nature an acid mucopolysaccharide and not a protein. Hence it follows that the precipitates in the canal system are not formed by the permeating liquid inside the bladder cavity. The main stems of the excretory canals of the bladder wall and of the invaginated portion were also packed and dilated, the canals being mostly filled with a homogeneous, highly PAS positive precipitate. The tissues, although necrotic, retained their shape and coloured with acidophilic stains. In the entrance canal a thin cuticular layer with a rim of surface extension was tearing away from the surface of the folds; later, the cuticle disappeared also from the invaginated canal. After the bladder had shrivelled and the necrotic parasite was permeated with serous exudate, most of its characteristic features were eliminated. The whole focus stained red with Goldner, yellow with van Gieson. Sometimes, the autolyzed tissue stained red with Goldner and could then be again partly demonstrated on the green background (Plate XXVI, Fig. 1). In such instances it is possible to study the structure of the parasite in sections impregnated with Gomori's method, in which the connective tissue skeleton and thus also the characteristic microscopical structure of the parasite can surprizingly often be viewed unless it has been destroyed by the tissue reaction of the scarring focus (Plate XVI, Fig. 1 and 2). Calcareous corpuscles disappeared very early during autolysis, sometimes leaving only empty spaces. Often, however, the proteinic skeleton of these formations persisted in the necrotic tissue and the corpuscles were the first site in which calcium was deposited during the dystrophic calcification. In such cases these skeletons could be demonstrated even in decalcified sections with Giemsa (dark violet); with alum haematoxylin they stained as sites of calcium deposition (Plate XVI, Fig. 3). The dystrophic calcification of the remnants of the parasite's tissue and of the exudate, sometimes forming only minute foci in the connective tissue scar, develop through the bond of calcium to the proteinic component consisting of grains of different sizes. In decalcified sections these grains could also be demonstrated with Giemsa and haematoxylin but should not be mistaken for remnants of the calcareous corpuscles especially as some of these have a concentric structure and are often of large size (Plate XVI, Fig. 4). Also disintegrating artifacts could be observed in a necrotic cysticercus, shaped like vacuoles with a remarkably differentiated surface layer and containing acid mucopolysaccharides. Such formations were frequently present in the cavity of the invaginated canal or at the opening of the ducts on the surface of the folds. The structure of the folded wall of the invaginated canal, the suckers, the rostellum and fragments of the bladder wall could nearly always be demonstrated with Gomori's method even in completely calcified foci. The hooks of the cysticercus, not being resorbed even after enclosure in the giant cells, were sometimes found directly in the hyaline connective tissue (Plate XXVI, Fig. 5). Stained selectively with Giemsa, they could be demonstrated equally well in areas of necrosis (Plate XXVI, Fig. 2), in the calcified focus and in the minute connective tissue scar. Their discovery is the irrefutable evidence of the presence of the cysticercus.

All these special examination methods should be performed on complete series of histological sections (see ŠLAIS 1960, 1968) to obtain reliable results when examining a suspicious focus. The importance of this procedure can be demonstrated by the results obtained by GIBSON (1959) who, using only routine histological methods, detected fragments of C. bovis in only 3 out of the 18 degenerated cysts examined. Particularly in human muscles, calcified suspected foci can be detected with x-rays, but sometimes these findings are only incidental. SIGMUND (1927) demonstrated them after 33 and 26 years following the outbreak of the acute form of the disease, PETROVICKY (1956) after 28 years, but none of these findings was confirmed histologically. WEISER (1942) studied the differential x-ray diagnosis of cysticercosis. GELASIUS (1962) studying the cysticercus of the cestode *Hydatigera taeniaeformis* demonstrated the rapid deposition of calcium salts during the degeneration of the bladder, some parts of which became calcified even before the death of the larva. The fact that in contrast to other cysticercus species even the bladder of the *Sc. fasciolaris* contains many calcareous corpuscles, explains the apparent anomaly of our observations of a dystrophic calcification affecting mainly the parenchymatous portion of the parasite and not its bladder.

## 4.   Differential diagnosis of various cysticercus species in man

The cysticercus species which is responsible for an infection of man may be identified by morphological studies. However, until now, no detailed study of this problem has been available because material has been relatively scarce and examination methods of the parasites, generally at an advanced stage of autolysis and resorption, are most difficult. The easiest to identify is a cysticercus with and invaginated scolex, in which, after evagination, the presence of hooks indicates *C. cellulosae* and their absence *C. bovis*. However, it is very important to remember that in cysticercal forms with an outgrown scolex the first sign of degeneration of the parasite is the loss of hooks from the rostellum (Plate XI, Fig. 1). Hooks in the exudative fluid permeating the formation fall mainly into the folds of the wall of the invaginated portion, where we discovered them repeatedly. However, the scolex retains its shape and in diagnosis, particularly if only a total mount is available, this scolex may be erronously mistaken for an unarmed one evaginated by pressure. Only an examination of a complete series of histological sections may ensure the identification of the hooks even after the complete resorption of the parasite in the hyaline connective tissue of the scar (Plate XXVI, Fig. 5).

In cerebral cysticercosis of man, the recovered scolex should be differentiated from the larval stage of the cestode *Multiceps multiceps* (LESKE, 1780) which causes coenurosis. The character of its cysts is, however, different; they are generally larger in size, their wall contains numerous invaginated scolices and the hooks are of a smaller size. So far, this disease has been recorded mainly from South Africa (70% of all described cases — after ROBINSON 1962), predominantly from areas of extensive sheep breeding, because *Coenurus cerebralis* develops mainly in the brain of these animals. A single, confirmed case of coenurosis in man was described by CORREA et al. (1962) from South America. Some reports on the incidence of this infection have come from Mexico (CABALLERO 1959). BRICENO et al. (1961) and BIAGI and BRICENO (1961) describing 97 cases of cysticercosis of man in Mexico drew attention to the relatively high incidence of infection with the racemose cysticercus (25%), considering in fact the possibility of another cysticercus than *C. cellulosae* being responsible for the origin of the racemose form. Sporadic reports of this infection have also been available from the United States, from Spain and England, where BICKERSTAFF (1955) raised the question about the etiology of solitary, intraventricular cysts and racemose cysts in association with basal meningo-encephalitis. Isolated findings of coenurosis have also been recorded from France (BRUMPT 1913, HOGER et al. 1942, DUPLAY et al. 1955). There, also, another species, *Coenurus serialis*, was found in man, although this species is known to develop in the muscles of the rabbit (e.g. BONNAL et al. 1933, BRUMPT et al. 1934).

When a scolex is found, the coenurus can be identified by the shape and the number of the hooks. Scolices are generally very numerous particularly in the advanced stage of development of the parasite. In this way most of the findings from South Africa have been confirmed (BECKER and JACOBSON 1951, WATSON and LAURIE 1955, WAINRIGHT 1957). The fact that young cysts of the coenurus, which frequently settle at the base of the brain before starting to grow directly in the ventricles and the cerebral parenchyma, have their scolices not yet developed, made BECKER and JACOBSON (1951) believe that all racemose and grapelike cysts of parasitic origin, especially those found in the posterior skull cavity, are of coenurus origin. DUPLAY et al. (1955) pointed out that these authors added to their observations a number of parasitologically unconfirmed and incompletely described cases merely because they were discovered in a sheep rearing area. Also BICKERSTAFF et al. (1956) maintained that when a racemose cysticercus occurred in the posterior skull cavity it was often possible to find typical cysticerci in other sections of the brain and that the coenurus cysts were not of a normal racemose appearance. However, without finding a scolex it would be most difficult to differentiate a coenurus bladder from a racemose cysticercus at an advanced stage when a resorptive tissue reaction had occurred as pointed out by ANGULA and ROQUE (1948). For this reason the histological structure of the bladder wall is of such importance. If its histological structure is retained the cysticercus species can, under favourable conditions, be identified (Plate XVII).

The possibility of identifying the parasite by its bladder is of great importance for the differential diagnosis of *C. cellulosae* and *Coenurus cerebralis* in the racemose form of cerebral cysticercosis. In addition to the typical subcuticular muscles in the bladder wall of *C. cellulosae* which, when contracted, are responsible for the wartlike surface of the cuticle, there are also differences in the protrusions on the surface of the bladder wall. In *Coenurus cerebralis* this rugate surface was observed only in parasites fixed after their extirpation from the brain. When in situ the coenurus wall is rather smooth and in older, larger cysts mostly extremely expanded, as is characteristic of this parasite. The protrusions are similar in character to those in *C. bovis* although smaller in size (28—46 µm wide at the base, 15—22 µm high). Therefore, in size they more closely resemble *C. cellulosae*, while their height to width index of 0·46 indicates a folded surface of the wall similar to that in *C. bovis*.

Moreover, there is another difference becoming particularly marked in a bladder which has starting to autolyze. Very often we observed a state in which the surface layers were separated from the main parenchymatous portion of the wall by large artificial interstices. Responsible for this state was the abnormally developed, more superficially situated system of wide canals lying close under the subcuticular layer. Generally, these canals attain a width of up to 40 µm while at the crossing points the lacunae measure even 120 µm in diameter. In this respect the width of the thin canals of the bottom network is in keeping with that of other cysticerci. These abnormally large lumina of the canals of the more superficially located network could be seen even in an extremely expanded wall. Under unfavourable osmotic conditions, these abnormally dilated canals disturb the homogeneity of the wall and separate the proper parenchymatous portion, which is relatively solid. Sometimes, this abnormal dilation of the canals of the more superficially situated network can be found also in *C. cellulosae* and *C. bovis* but, in view of the localization of these cysticerci, this tends rather to destroy the parenchymatous portion of the wall instead of separating it from the cuticle and the subcuticular layer as in *Coenurus cerebralis*. The height of the very fine extensions on the surface of the cuticle of *Coenurus cerebralis* is about 1 µm and never exceeds 2 µm. No calcareous corpuscles are present in the parenchyma of its wall except round the openings of the invaginate scolices.

Although the identification of *C. bovis* in the brain of man has not conclusively been confirmed, this species has been included in table 3 together with *C. cellulosae*, *Coenurus cerebralis* and also the echinococcus, the bladder of this last having been described from the brain of man.

BRUMPT (1949) saw a difference between the bladder of *C. cellulosae* and that of *Coenurus cerebralis*. In the wall of *C. cerebralis* the protrusions were bigger and were called by him papillae. He believed that the hairlike processes of the surface of the cuticle originated from its dissociation. He maintained that they are considerably smaller than those of the larva of *T. solium*, a conclusion with which we agree. Also WAINRIGHT (1957) in an attempt to differentiate histologically the typical *C. cellulosae*, the racemose form of the cerebral cysticercus and the coenurus found that variations in the "papillary folds" and hairlike projections could not be used for specific differentiation. Variations could occur in one and the same cyst. He drew attention to the possible variability of these features in relation to age and tension of cyst. In his opinion the specific origin of the racemose cyst could be confirmed only if scolices also were found. Our findings, however, suggest the possibility of a histological differentiation of these cysticercus species.

Of the other cerebral parasites, solitary echinococcus cysts can be identified reliably by the stratified, hyaloidine membrane on the surface of the parasite's bladder. The cerebral changes caused by paragonimiasis, an infection endemic in East and Southeast Asia, are very different in nature. A recent description given by STEFANKO and ŽEBROWSKI (1961) from Korea showed the main features to be the formation of pseudocysts and the granulomatous reaction to the eggs of this trematode.

When identifying histologically necrotic and calcified formations localized in other organs of man than the brain it is possible to demonstrate not only hooks but also other cuticular sclerites such as fanglike linguatula hooks or even fragments of the cuticle of nematodes. Most resistant to resorption are also the coverings of the eggs of the parasite which may be found in parasitic granulomas. We described

Table 3.

Diagnostic characters of some cestode larvae which may be found in man

| | | C. cellulosae | C. bovis | Coenurus cerebralis | Echinococcus granulosus |
|---|---|---|---|---|---|
| Scolex | | 1 | 1 | several | many |
| Hooks | | + | 0 | + | + |
| Bladder | surface | cuticle | cuticle | cuticle | stratified hyaloidine membrane |
| | superficial hairlike cuticular extensions | ranging from below 1 μm to 2·5 μm | 3—6 μm | 1—2 μm | 0 |
| | subcuticular groups of muscles | + | 0 | 0 | 0 |
| | make-up of wall surface | wartlike processes | rugae | smooth and also rugate | smooth |
| | base of superficial protuberances | 27—38 μm | 50—70 μm | 28—46 μm | 0 |
| | height of superficial protuberances | 15—27 μm | 23—27 μm | 15—22 μm | 0 |

several methods of identification of the parasite in some earlier papers (ŠLAIS 1960, 1962, 1962/63, 1963, 1964a,b). During an exhaustive and systematic examination of minute, mostly calcified foci localized generally under the capsule of the liver, we discovered also necrotic formations without resistant sclerites which, in view of their symmetrical, histological structure could hardly have been mere artifacts (ŠLAIS 1966).

At one end of a striped, hyaline node we discovered in the necrotic centre the oval section of a formation with a central cavity, its wall being permeated with vacuoles of different sizes. Its surface could still be stained red with van Gieson's method. With Goldner's method it was possible to distinguish in this superficial layer thin, red-staining stripes, extending through the green surface layer. These stripes stained bluish-violet with Mallory's phosphotungstic haematoxylin and traversed at right angles. The minute cell nuclei of different size in the tissue under the surface with diameters of only one half or even less of that of the nearby nuclei of the exudate and liver cells also were stainable. Silver staining after Gomori revealed that the necrotic exudate was interspersed with fibres of the newly formed connective tissue which, being also necrotic, radiated from the surface of the necrosis to its centre. In this method, a marked surface layer of reticular nature could be seen on this central formation (Plate XVIII, Fig. 2), from which fibrils radiated to its central cavity. The border-line of the central cavity consisted of a system of coarse, interlaced fibres enclosing a system of canals with lumina of different width. The largest measurements of the oval section of this suspected formation were: height 420 μm, width 600 μm. Its third dimension estimated from the number of histological sections in the series was about 400—700 μm. The central cavity measured 120 μm in height, 270 μm in width, the surrounding wall being 120 μm thick. The staining properties of the tissue fragment thus showed that the formation was covered with a thin, limiting layer, which was followed by a network of muscle fibres lying at right angles in a substance of connective tissue nature. The radial arrangement of the fibrils under this layer and also the bordering of the central cavity suggested a histologically differentiated wall of a young cysticercus larva with a system of fibres and canals. The apparent vacuolization of the wall was in keeping with the dilated canal system. Also the size and shape of the demonstrable remnants of cell nuclei suggested the parenchyma of lower worms. The whole formation could, therefore, be classified as the early stage of a cysticercus with a differentiating central body cavity and a body wall.

In the central cavity of the homogeneous exudate of the second node we found a spherical, solid formation 180 μm in diameter (Plate XVIII, Fig. 1). On its surface we distinguished a fine, limiting layer and under it a layer of connective tissue containing muscle fibres. Under the surface layer minute cell nuclei were concentrated; towards the centre, these were considerably less dense resembling reticular tissue. The centre of the formation was filled with material of an indefinable nature. Adjacent to the surface of the formation and also to the remaining periphery of the cavity there was a strongly staining, wrinkled membrane.

At first, the etiology of this undefined, spherical formation was obscure, but after comparing it with the formation found in the earlier observation, it could clearly be identified as the young developmental stage of a cysticercus with a differentiating central body cavity and body wall.

On the grounds of their histological structure it was possible to demonstrate that the two minute, necrotic formations found in the liver of man were early developmental stages (mother bladders) of a cestode larva — the cysticercus. Evidently, these cysticerci showed an affinity for the liver. Although *C. cellulosae and C. bovis* may be found exceptionally in these organs, in this case it was not possible to consider them to be either of these two species. Their unusual occurrence in the liver is connected generally with a high incidence in other organs. Particularly in our first observation there was clear evidence that this cysticercus pierced marked, destructive passages into the parenchyma of the organ. Therefore, we had to exclude the possibility of confusion with *Sc. fasciolaris*, which settles and develops only in the liver. Moreover, a thin-walled bladder originating from the oncosphere is formed very early after the parasite has settled in the liver and these bladders are completely different from the ones we found. Thus, these could only have been cysticerci which passed through the liver on their way to the abdominal cavity to complete their development. In Czechoslovakia, a possible species would be *C. pisiformis*, normally developing in rabbits and hares. This species, however, forms a central cavity at a later stage, when the elongate larva has attained a length of 4—5 mm and, by that time, has generally left the liver. Thus it seemed necessary to consider the parasite to be *C. tenuicollis*, the cysticercus of the cestode *T. hydatigena*, which commonly develops in the abdominal cavity of various domestic animals. We compared our findings from the liver of man with young cysticerci obtained from artificial and natural, massive *C. tenuicollis* infestations of the liver of lamb and swine (Plate XVIII, Fig. 3 and 4). In spite of the necrotic and autolytic changes we were almost certain of their identity with *C. tenuicollis*. Our findings show that cysticerci can develop in man when he is a completely atypical host, this occurring, for example, in an infection with eggs of *T. hydatigena* and other cestodes. However, the larvae, having settled in an abnormal host, are killed abruptly by the defence reaction and cannot complete their development.

## 5. Mistakes in the diagnosis of cysticercosis in pathology

Mistakes in the diagnosis of a cysticercosis are quite common not only because the parasite is mistaken for another affection, which, in view of its necrosis and disintegration, is quite understandable, but also because some structures of the parasite are misinterpreted and give rise to injudicious theories. Most common is the misinterpretation of calcareous corpuscles for the eggs of the parasite, although their morphology has been well-known since the times of Virchow. GALLAIS et al. (1955) describing the bladder of a cerebral cysticercus, which could have been easily identified on the evidence of their own photomicrographs, believed the remnant of the invaginated canal of the parasite, found in the focus of necrosis, to be part of the uterus and the staining skeleton of the calcareous corpuscles to be even embryonated eggs. This suggested to them the finding of a special cerebral nematode, which they tried to identify and to arrange in its systematic position. KUFS (1951, 1952), studying a case of massive cerebral cysticercosis, misinterpreted the calcareous corpuscles in the parenchyma of the young stages of the parasite for unfertilized eggs; because these are one of the last structures starting to differentiate in the cysticercus, he discovered them at various developmental stages. From this erroneous identification he deduced his new theory about the development of the eggs in the larva; moreover, he misidentified the scolex as an embryonic centre similar to a proglottid. Although this completely erroneous theory was criticized by SCHMIDT - HOENSDORF and PETZENBURG (1958), other authors such as RABL (1958) and PIAZZA and GADDO (1962) still referred to it. Rabl observed in his case of a meningeal cysticercosis some formations in the necrotic remnants of the cysticercus which, under the influence of Kufs' theory, he identified as various developmental stages of other cysticerci. His photomicrographs show quite clearly that these formations are disintegrating artifacts of the necrotic exudate with calcium deposits particularly in the surface layer of these spherical structures, similar to those observed by us in a number of cases. The deposition of calcium salts is responsible for the remarkable staining properties of this surface layer. Tangential sections of these disintegrating vacuoles were mistaken by this author for vital structures. Also his conclusion that a high incidence of cysticerci in the brain is mostly accompanied by a locally originating infection, is completely unsubstantiated.

The differential diagnosis of the cerebral cysticercus, especially in a stage of necrosis, from nonparasitic affections may be most difficult particularly when the material is incomplete. Here, it is important to differentiate epidermoid cysts and tumors causing similar obstructive symptoms as do the cysticerci especially in the brain chambers. Necrotic masses of cholesteatome are often spherical in shape; also the encapsulating connective tissue becomes dystrophically calcified resembling calcified cysts which, when of larger size, might be mistaken for an echinococcus. GOTFRÝD et al. (1958) erroneously identified necrotic hair follicles and sebaceous glands as cysticercus structures, although the formation was actually an intracranial dermoid. Also solitary meningeal foci being either calcified or ossified, need a detailed histological analysis to demonstrate their parasitic origin. In such instances it is necessary to bear in mind mainly the ossification of the Pacchionian bodies and a local metastatic calcification of the meninges, but sometimes their etiology cannot be revealed. The definite proof of the cysticercus is the finding of hooks in minute scars in the brain during the examination of serial sections. When making a differential diagnosis of the racemose cysticercus, particularly when localized at the base of the brain, we found it necessary to differentiate macroscopically similar bladders originating in an arachnoiditis cystica and the lobate formation of an ossifying lipoma.

MARTINEC and GUILIANI (1959) described a fatal case of bronchopneumonia in a 37 year-old women after operation. In the lungs, they found spherical to ovoid corpuscles, measuring from 100—250 µm, which they considered to be early larval stages "cysticercoids" of cestodes of the family Cyclophilloidea and the etiological agent of the disease. According to these writers autolysis was so advanced that exact identification was impossible. Some observations on the same pseudoparasitic formations were described in Slovakia and, having been consulted in one case, we identified these findings as plant tissue. Also DLUHOŠ et al. (1962) demonstrated an observation of a similar, giant-cell granuloma in the lungs of a child, which was erroneously identified as being of mycotic origin. CROME and VALENTINE (1962) showed that similar corpuscles may be a secondary finding in the lungs later evoking even a giant cell- and histiocytic reaction. These were aspirated single cells especially from edible seeds of leguminous crops. VIDVARTHI (1967) came to the same conclusions.

## 6. Diagnosis and research on muscle cysticercosis of cattle and on taeniarhynchosis of man

The increasing incidence of muscle cysticercosis in cattle has centered the interests of veterinarians on this disease. In Europe, numerous communications have been published on this problem and information has been available from Austria (KEIBEL 1961), Switzerland (DESPRÉS 1962), the Netherlands (HONER 1963) and elsewhere. Attempts of the veterinarians to control this infection have sometimes been directed towards the problem of the time of survival of the cysticerci in the carcasses (KOVALEV 1965), but are mainly concerned with improving diagnostic methods used for the detection of bovine cysticercosis at abattoirs. DEWHIRST et al. (1967) analyzed the incidence of bovine cysticercosis in the United States and estimated the effectivity of current inspection procedures for detecting bovine cysticercosis. They concluded that antemortem tests were better for detecting the infection than current inspection of carcasses. Of practical importance are interdermal and hemagglutination tests. For the application of these methods, the preparation of the antigen is of utmost importance. At present, the best results seem to have been achieved with a natural antigen, with which KOSMINKOV (1965) reported obtaining positive results in 41·3%. This author maintained that an antigen obtained with biochemical methods from the scolices of *C. bovis* is less effective. In a more recent report KOSMINKOV and FILIPPOV (1967) recommended the use of a polystyrene latex in serological reactions for the diagnosis of bovine cysticercosis. SOKOLOVSKAYA and MOSKVIN (1967) proved that this antigen produced by this method from cysticerci was more suitable for identifying the cysticercus than an extract from mature segments of the adult cestode.

An important factor in the infection of cattle with cysticercosis is the susceptibility of the animals and, in this respect, the relationship of sex to infection, which was confirmed by KOUDELA (1966) is most interesting. The marked incidence in oxen in comparison with other groups is quite evident from Koudela's report and particularly noteworthy in the arrangement of the material into age groups. At present, the explanation of this phenomenon is only hypothetical. Live and regressively changed parasites in the infected animals, studied at the same time, showed a certain organ specificity, most of the degenerating cysts having been found in the heart. The non-uniform course and intensity of reaction to *C. bovis* in muscle cysticercosis seems to depend in the first place on the number of oncospheres causing the infection. A particularly high incidence in calves, as described by Leuckart in his experiments, led to a generalized infection and to a macroscopic picture of milliary tuberculosis with calcified cysts and undeveloped parasites. Another important question is acquired immunity, because the dependence of the course of tissue reaction to the parasite to the age of the animal has been proved repeatedly (KOUDELA 1967). The predominance of regressively changed cysticerci over the live ones is very marked in the higher age groups especially in animals older than 8 years. This suggests that the concurrent appearance of live and regressively changed cysticerci does not necessarily indicate an acute reinfection as was confirmed by HILLER (1941). Records are available of relatively increased numbers of regressively changed parasites at times of a high or maximum incidence of bovine cysticercosis. Numerous investigators have also attempted by experimental research work to find an answer to the problem of active immunity and its origin.

One of the centres of research work on bovine cysticercosis was Kenya, where investigations into the frequency of cysticercosis (FROYD 1960) were followed by research work performed by URQUHART (1961) who observed that calves soon after birth are most susceptible, becoming infected generally in the first weeks of life. This natural infection is usually characterized by a low incidence of cysts, their localization and developmental stage suggesting that the infection occurred on the day of birth or soon after. Even artificial prenatal infection could not be demonstrated. In the author's opinion, a resistance due to active immunity may be accompanied by an innate individual resistance. Both these factors seem thus responsible for the high resistance of the calves to artificial infection so that in some animals in the experiment it was not possible to demonstrate cysticerci from an artificial infection, while in others only undeveloped cysts and an advanced tissue reaction were found. A comparison with the experiments performed on calves in Scotland revealed that these were not actively immune and that the incidence of parasites following the artificial infection, was very high. FROYD and ROUND (1959) and FROYD (1961) infected artificially adult bovines with hatched oncospheres of *Trh. saginatus* by injecting them subcutaneously. The larvae, however, developed only locally into adult cysticerci without any influence on a natural or artificial oral infection. It is interesting that in some cows the larvae moved into the local lymph-glands and developed there into cysticerci, this supporting our view that the cysticercus is a parasite of the lymphatic vessel system. The described experiment suggested the possibility that in a parenteral infection the cysticerci can develop even in bovine animals with a well developed immunity to oral infection. Therefore, ROUND (1961) considered the possible role played by blood-sucking flies as vectors of bovine cysticercosis in East Africa, because there the cattle are known to possess a well developed immunity to oral infection. URQUHART (1965) had some doubts about the importance of parenteral transmission of cysticercosis in greatly infested, enzootic regions maintaining that the flies could transmit only eggs but not hatched oncospheres, only with which the experiments were successful.

The occurrence of immunity in artificially infected calves was also confirmed by LEIKINA et al. (1964) who found not only a greatly restricted reinfection, but a considerable shortening of the viability of cysticerci from the second and even from the first infection. FROYD (1963) was unsuccessful in his attempt to prepare a highly specific antigen for intradermal use in cattle infected with cysticercosis. Similarly until the present it has not been possible to confirm cysticercosis with the dermal test as tried by GRABER and THOME (1964) in the Central African republic Chad because there is a cross reaction of this test with various trematodes and cestodes. These authors drew attention also to the different epizootological situation in bovine cysticercosis in this region compared with that in Kenya explaining this mainly on the basis of different climatic conditions. LUCKER and VEGORS (1965) demonstrated in their experimental animals that the cysticerci from X-ray irradiated cestode eggs develop considerably slower. Despite this, they found a distinct immunity in the animals infected with these eggs in a preliminary experiment.

GEMMEL (1962) in an attempt to find an answer to the specificity of antibody in the individual cysticercus species pointed out two important components participating in the origin of immunity: the early response during the passage of the oncosphere through the intestinal barrier which, in his opinion, is more significant than the second response during the development of the cysticercus at the site of its localization. GEMMEL (1965a) vaccinated rabbits with either live eggs or hatched oncospheres of *T. pisiformis*, *T. ovis* and *T. hydatigena*, infecting them afterwards perorally with eggs of *T. pisiformis*. The injected eggs and larvae of *T. pisiformis* evoked a relatively good immunity to natural infection with this cestode, this being exhibited particularly during the passage of the larvae through the liver and during the establishment and continuance of the larvae in the omentum of the experimental animals. A certain resistance to a natural infection with *C. pisiformis* was exhibited even after an injection with hatched larvae of the other two cestodes but not after an injection of their eggs. In later experiments GEMMEL (1965b) found that a good immunity against *T. ovis* can be obtained also in sheep vaccinated with activated embryos of this species and, to a lesser degree, also with the eggs. A certain immunity against the development of cysticerci of this species was obtained with activated embryos of *T. hydatigena*, while the immunity was practically nil after injecting activated embryos of *T. pisiformis*. The results of these cross experiments suggest a certain relationship between *T. ovis* and *T. hydatigena*. These results are most difficult to explain and the properties of the hosts should be considered the main factor, the sheep being a host of both *T. ovis* and *T. hydatigena*, the rabbit only of *T. pisiformis*. GEMMEL believed the active and passive immunity to be conditioned by the antibody produced particularly against the metabolic products of the larva during its metamorphosis and not against the somatic antigens of the parasitic embryos. The greater success of a homologous vaccination with activated embryos may also explain their better chance of a normal development than that is the case with injected eggs. Gemmel's findings, however, cannot be applied to other cysticerci as shown by similar, but unsuccessful attempts by FROYD (1961) to evoke immunity against *C. bovis* in cattle by injecting activated embryos of this species. The use of immunofluorescent methods in research on cysticercosis is still in its initial stage because it is difficult to distinguish the nature of specific and unspecific fluorescence especially in the calcareous corpuscles in the parenchyma of the parasite.

The attention paid to bovine cysticercosis is not only based on economic factors but also on its epidemiological importance. The incidence of infection of man with *Trh. saginatus* in Europe has been steadily increasing in the last ten years according to the literature. Under good hygienic conditions of Central Europe, great attention has been given to this relatively important parasitosis. In Czechoslovakia diagnostic methods and the clinical treatment of taeniarhynchosis has been studied by PETRŮ et al. (1966) and others. The problem of the carriers of this cestode as a source of constant infection of cattle in certain areas is being investigated by REHNOVÁ (1967). The increasing incidence of this infection in Central Europe is in direct relationship to the increasing popularity of dishes made of raw beef. In countries where similar dishes are common, closed communicties may become highly infected with this cestode. In two district of Azerbaidzhan, the infestation rate of the population with the cestode *Trh. saginatus* was 4·5 and 17%, but according to ABASOV (1965) the introduction of effective control measures eliminated it in 2—3 years. Also in other central Asian areas of the U.S.S.R. (MAGDIEV et al. 1965) and in the Ukraine (SHULMAN and KAMINSKIY 1964) the control of taeniarhynchosis is of the greatest interest. In Poland, great attention has been paid to the serological diagnosis of this disease. MACHNICKA - ROGUSKA and ZWIERZ (1964) using the haemagglutination test concluded that a positive finding depends directly on the presence of the parasite and symptoms disappear very quickly after its removal. MACHNICKA - ROGUSKA (1965) made an exhaustive, biochemical analysis of an antigen prepared from *Trh. saginatus.* Later MACHNICKA - ROGUSKA and ZWIERZ (1966) demonstrated that, in the haemagglutination test, the polysaccharide fraction of the antigen is the most active one while in the complement fixation test this is the protein-nucleoproteinic fraction. A comparison of antigen prepared from the cysticercus with that from the adult cestode will be of great importance for immunological studies of cysticercosis.

# Pathogenicity of *Cysticercus cellulosae* and *Cysticercus bovis*

## 1. Tissue reaction in muscle cysticercosis caused by *Cysticercus cellulosae*

In a massive, acute muscle cysticercosis of swine we observed only minimal changes in the tissues surrounding the parasites in spite of the large number of viable parasites which already had fully developed bladders. The connective tissue wall of the lymphatic space was very thin (15—20 µm) especially at the sites adjoining the adipose tissue and lacked the arrangement of collageneous fibrils in its crossing layers. The thicker parts of the wall (up to 50 µm and above) seemed to be the dilated crossing points of the lymphatic capillary network, in which connective tissue had concentrated, because we often found a direct transition into the undilated part. In it the original lumen of the capillary was slitshaped and winding. A nodular concentration of connective tissue indicated the site of attachment of the larger bundles of muscle fibres, attenuating in spindle fashion and terminating in it (Plate XIII, Fig. 1, Plate XIV). In the musculature of bovine animals, however, these muscle fibre bundles are attached to the stronger partitions, their connective tissue especially that of the larger bundles being more like tendons. Although similar lamellae may also be present in the musculature of swine, in them they are very thin and loose.

The nodularly concentrated connective tissue in swine is also less organized and contains more cells. The greater concentration of cells suggests the presence of infiltration cells. Minute foci of accumulated infiltration cells were observed only exceptionally, sometimes even at the thin wall limiting the cysticercus. Between the wall of the bladder and the surface of the lymphatic space we found solitary, rounded cells of histiocytic appearance, sometimes arranged in a single layer. Only quite exceptionally were they more densely packed, appearing like effused exudate. Sometimes, a lymphoid infiltration was found at the periphery of the focus, but only in one parasite did this resembled small lymphatic follicles similar to those originating in a reaction to *C. bovis*. Topographically, however, being situated at the pointed termination of the bladder, this had no connection with the opening of the invaginated canal. Also once only did we note an indistinct, coagulated exudative liquid between the bladder of the parasite and the wall as the only sign of tissue reaction found in our ample material.

Parasites of a typically elongate shape from a cysticercosis of the human diaphragm were calcified, lying freely in a thick encapsulation of connective tissue parallel to the course of the muscle bundles. The nodules occupied almost the whole breadth of the diaphragm. The layer of encapsulating connective tissue measured approximately 150 µm. The fibroblasts on the inner side of the encapsulation resembled younger, settling cells, forming the surface of an encapsulation without any other lining. On the outer side of the capsule only minimal signs of the infiltrate were found near the vessels, extending between the encapsulation and the musculature. In their vicinity we found solitary, plasmatic cells and forms of cell nuclei indicating a through- passage of exudate cells. The histological character of the encapsulation was almost analogous to that surrounding the cysticerci in the meninges of the cerebellum in this observation.

In the generalized cysticercosis of man we found most of the parasites localized in the skeletal muscles, discovering, however, only necrotic and calcified remnants in a thick, hyaline connective tissue capsule, which often was also partly calcified. In the roentgenographic diagnosis of the cysticercosis the foci resembled the no longer existing bladder of the parasite only in their oval and ovoid shape. In all cysts it was possible to demonstrate unresorbed remnants of the parasites; hooks were often found in a hyaline, connective tissue encapsulation. Their advanced age at the time of their death was confirmed by the many findings of outgrown scolices of the cysticerci. The hyaline capsule was often surrounded by adipose tissue and atrophied muscle fibres. Tissue reaction in the vicinity of the parasitic remnants indicated the very long period, perhaps many years, elapsing since the actual outbreak of the disease. The most prominent formation discovered at the site of attachment of the papillary muscle to the endocardium contained calcified remnants of a cysticercus with an outgrown scolex enclosed in a thick hyaline encapsulation. In its vicinity also the endocardium was greatly thickened. In this unusual finding in the human heart the parasitic cyst localized under the endocardium did not break through but only bulged to a great extent into the heart chamber.

## 2.  Tissue reaction in cysticercosis of the meninges and the brain tissue

There is little knowledge available on the early changes in cerebral cysticercosis of man, because the pathological picture of the disease becomes revealed mostly at a much later stage. Solitary cysts in symptomatically unresponding sites are only incidental post mortem findings, but even a multiple cysticercosis may be very advanced before causing the death of the infected person, because the greatest tissue reaction sets in during the decomposition of the parasite. It has repeatedly been confirmed that there is hardly any reaction to the growing cysticercus, which affects the surrounding tissue only by its pressure as a slowly growing formation.

While studying material from a multiple cysticercosis we discovered a shrivelled, parasitic bladder being trapped by the encapsulating reaction in the fissura lateralis cerebri at the site where it touched the activated meninges (Fig. 25). Only once did we discover an atrophy of the cortex at a stage, in which only the disappearance of the neurons and the deposition of lipofuscine in the glial cells could be observed (Plate XIX, Fig. 1). Only few lymphocytes were found in the unchanged pial membrane. We also discovered several cysts without any signs of degeneration (Fig. 26) or with autolysis just starting and with an atrophy of the cortex in their vicinity. This was

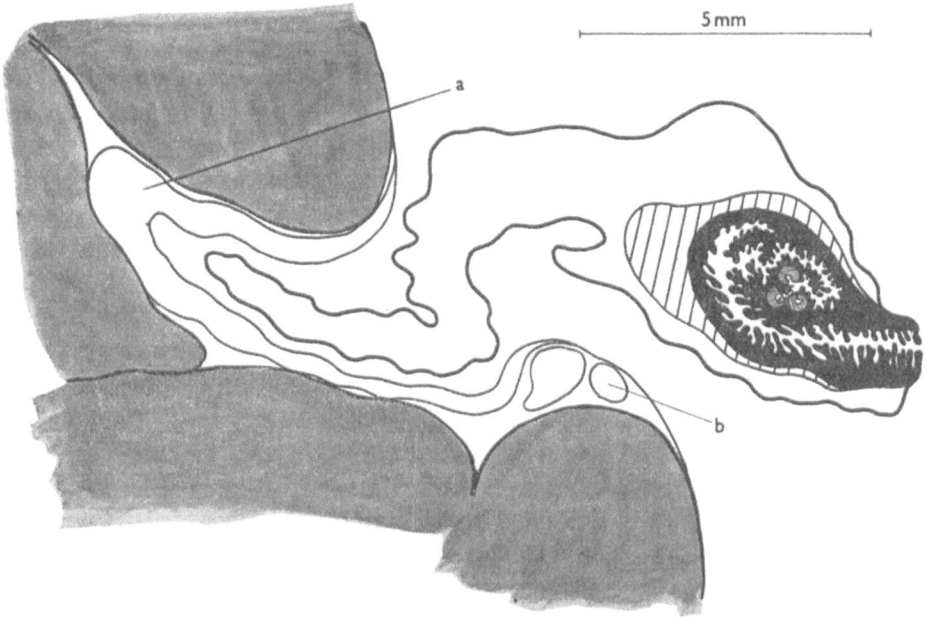

Fig. 25. Scheme illustrating the successive growth of the connective tissue encapsulation round the collapsed cysticercus at the surface of the brain. a — connective tissue, b — vessels.

characterized by a marked attenuation of the cortex, the disappearance of nerve cells and diffuse gliosis whereby the marginal layer of the glial fibres was not thickened.

Around several cysticerci, which were still uncollapsed and pressed into the gyri, it was possible to demonstrate the gradual development of tissue reaction. One of the poles was closely adjoining the pia, in which lymphocytes, lymphoid elements of a transitional type, plasmatic cell and solitary eosinophilic cells formed a slight, local infiltrate. On the surface of the atrophic cortex there persisted an adequate marginal layer of glial fibres, while coatlike infiltrates of lymphocytes were found round the vessels under the surface of the cortex. The second pole of the bladder was pushed away from the fibrous capsule by a necrotic exudate, the invaginated portion of the parasite was mostly necrotic, the meninges thickened, fibrous, interspersed with vessels; on the outer side of the capsule we found an infiltrate consisting of numerous lymphocytes and plasmocytes. Closeby, there were often remnants of the largely resorbed cysticercus. The gradual development of the tissue reaction could be observed on the periphery of such cysts (Plate XX).

These findings suggest that the live cyst, although growing for a long time, evokes at first only a feeble reaction of the adjoining pial membranes. Only when the bladders are well developed does the surrounding connective tissue start to thicken. In the early stage lymphocytes and lymphocytic elements of a transitional shape

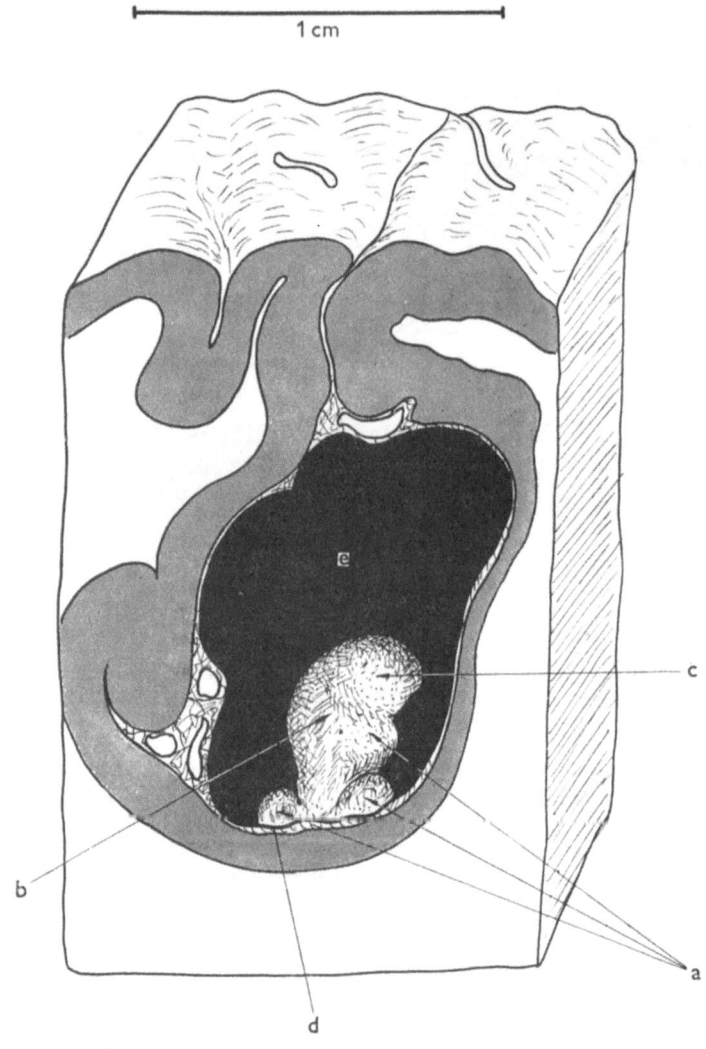

Fig. 26. Schematic diagram showing the localization of the cysticercus deep in the sulcus of the brain cortex. c — site of the invaginated portion in which the scolex is placed; b — site of the spiral and entrance canal; a — lobes of loosely arranged tissue adjoining the surface of the paren-chymatous portion of the brain cysticercus, characteristic of this form; d — connective tissue encapsulation; e — bladder cavity.

are found on the surface of the bladder. Mitoses of the activated fibroblasts were not discovered, but only young connective tissue elements, the amitotic formations of their nuclei and transitional forms of lymphocytic cells. Noteworthy are the shapes of the active exudative elements found during the formation of the connective tissue layer on the surface of the bladder, passing from the environment to its surface. The numbers of plasmocytes and their transitional forms from the lymphocytes also increase. The parasitic membrane was situated so close to the fine capsule especially at the site where its surface was folded in wartlike formations that, on the slides, it was not possible to distinguish the border between the cysticercus and the encapsulating tissue, in which the gradual maturation and fibrosis occurs.

Tissue reaction becomes distinctly increased after the death of the parasite is apparent. This, however, seems to be a very slow process. The first indication of metabolic changes is the stagnation of the liquid in the dilated system of excretory canals both in the bladder wall and in the invaginated portion. Coarser precipitates in the canals, reacting especially as mucopolysaccharides and proteins indicate the beginning of necrosis. This does not affect the whole bladder at once but starts at the invaginated portion spreading to the surrounding area. In an advanced autolysis of the central portion the cells of the more distant parts of the bladder wall still stain normally. This indicates that the development of tissue reaction around the parasite is not uniform.

In some places the accumulated, neutrophilic leukocytes separate the bladder wall from the fibrous encapsulation and this process continues along the periphery of the bladder wall. The cell exudate becomes necrotic and sometimes the necrosis affects even some parts of the connective tissue capsule. When the whole parasite has become necrotic, its bladder shrivels and serous exudate starts to fill the space between the connective tissue and the parasite. Exudate entering also into the invaginated canal, deforms and dilates it.

At a later stage gradual resorption sets in. Histiocytic cells proliferate on the outer surface of the fibrous encapsulation forming a loose, network-like layer containing giant cells. Multinucleate cells are liberated and enter also the exudate where they are resorbed in the same way as the parasitic tissue. Also the inner space with the accumulated exudate and the remnants of the cysticercus becomes reduced by the gradual retraction of the fibrous capsule. The remnants of the parasites adjoining the resorption border become destroyed by giant cells regardless of which structures of the parasite are concerned. Therefore, when examining the necrotic contents of a cyst it was not always possible to demonstrate the most typical features of the cysticercus. In the giant cells it were mainly the phagocytozed precipitates of the parasite's excretory canal system that could be detected, at this stage resembling some kind of pigment with special staining properties (see p. 92). This we showed also in the phagocytozing histiocytes of the fibrous capsule. In the greatly hyalinized capsule we found also other remnants of the resorbing parasite, especially the diagnostically important hooks. The resorption process is very slow. Sometimes, when the entire contents of the encapsulation have been resorbed a wrinkled hyaline scar with slits filled with loose connective tissue is formed. Hooks could always be detected in series of sections made of these scars, thus confirming the presence of a cysticercus. Sometimes, however, the remnants were calcified and dystrophic calcification affected also the hyaline capsule. In such instances even the specific structure of the parasite could be demonstrated.

In the vicinity of the resorption process the connective tissue is widely infiltrated with lymphocytes and plasmocytes, sporadically also with mast cells. No eosinophilic cells were detected at this stage. The intima of the vessels in the vicinity of the chronic inflammation is fibrously thickened, the elastic membrane is doubled or disturbed and the adventitia start to proliferate. The still persisting parts of the cortex are changed by gliosis, the connective tissue of the parasite's capsule radiates into the surrounding tissue and hemosiderinic pigment is deposited in the histiocytes. Near the scar most of the cortex disappears (Plate XIX, Fig. 2) and in the adjoining region of the white matter we discovered numerous macroglial elements forming a continuous rim between the white matter and the inflammatory connective tissue (Plate XX, Fig. 6). In the surface layer of the cortex and nearby, particularly in the white matter, we often detected numerous corpora amylacea. Even the infiltrate of lymphocytes and plasmocytes was almost absent in old, calcified, meningeal scars.

In a massive cysticercosis of the pia mater the meninges coalesce, thicken and become clouded. The encapsulated and resorbing bladders of the parasite appear through the meninges like well-defined, more solid and brownish nodules. In one of our observations the foci coalesced so firmly with the thickened meninges that they stuck to those removed from the surface of the brain like polypous formations torn away from the cortex. In all of them we discovered the invaginated portion of the parasite at an advanced stage of resorption. In another observation the cysts in the cerebellar meninges were so large that they always reached the white matter and disturbed the finer architecture of the nervous tissue much more than in the cerebrum (Plate XXV, Fig. 5); the tissue reaction, however, was still the same.

In a cysticercosis of the meninges it is generally possible to discover several cysts also in the brain matter. This is in agreement with the finding of solitary cysts in the meninges and the brain in muscle cysticercosis. A massive incidence inside the brain affects largely the course of the disease leading to early death. In our observation of an infection of this type the parasites attained only a young developmental stage and a small size, but the tissue reaction was greatly advanced. All parasites were surrounded by a relatively thick layer of fibrous connective tissue, its periphery being infiltrated with lymphocytes and plasmocytes. Only in some cysts did we discover the start of an exudate towards the inside. About one half of the parasites were found at different stages of calcification. Calcification affected first the calcareous corpuscles and the fibrous parenchyma of the invaginated portion, whereas the bladder still stained as a vital structure. This finding suggests the relatively high autonomy of growth of the bladder wall. At the sites where several parasites developed in close vicinity to each other, we discovered a necrosis of the scolex portion of one of them and necrotic exudate in its surroundings which, in view of the number of Charcot - Leyden crystals must have consisted mainly of eosinophilic leukocytes, which sometimes were still demonstrable. The connective tissue encapsulating the whole group also was necrotic and extended between the individual cysticerci like incomplete septa. It seems more likely that the strong tissue reaction and the necrosis of the parasite were due to the intense reaction of the host's organism and not to unfavourable conditions caused by a concentration of parasites in one place, because also in the musculature of swine cysticerci often develop in closely adjacent groups without impeding each other's development. The necrosis of the exudate and of the nearby connective tissue is caused by the direct contact with the dead necrotic parasites.

In a massive cysticercosis many cysts were localized so closely under the lining of the lateral cerebral ventricles that they bulged into them like peas. Several times we found the thin wall ruptured and in the opening a parasite as decribed above. In many places it was possible to demonstrate scars originating from these evacuated cavities (Plate XXVI, Fig. 3). Under the ependyma of the ventricles we also discovered glial nodules (ependymitis granularis). These changes, however, are not typical for cysticercosis. The ependymal lining of the bottom of the lateral ventricle above the greatly scarred cysticercus was quite normal.

Late tissue reaction round the individual parasites in the cerebral tissue is the same as that in the meninges. In the basal ganglia we discovered hyaline scars shaped like narrow stripes, measuring 2 − 3 mm on transverse section and containing minute remnants of exudate (Plate XXVI, Fig. 4). We considered their origin to be suggestive only because they were found in a cysticercus infected brain. The examination of complete series of histological sections revealed in them the hooks of the cysticercus suggesting that even in the brain tissue the completely developed cysticercus can be fully resorbed as in the musculature. Thereby, the glial scar was restricted only to a narrow rim round the connective tissue encapsulation. Since such advanced resorption is abnormal it cannot occur unless the necrotic contents have become dystrophically calcified. In two solitary cysts in the brain we found that the hyaline connective tissue capsule in the thick, glial scar changed into a lamellar bone containing fat marrow which indicated that the process must have lasted for very many years. Nevertheless it was possible to demonstrate remnants of parasitic structures in the calcified contents.

## 3.  Tissue reaction in muscle cysticercosis of cattle

The completely developed *C. bovis* with its invaginated portion in the bladder cavity lies at first in the dilated lymphatic space without evoking any tissue reaction.

Sometimes, precipitates of a finely granular character, which stain like proteins, are deposited directly on them. Cell elements are not present in these precipitates. The lining of the dilated space consists of a thin layer of flat cells with oval, elongate nuclei, measuring 18—20 μm in length and 6 μm in breadth (Plate XV, Fig. 3). The nuclei with a looser chromatin distribution contain several coarser granules with staining nucleoli which are of such negligible thickness that, in transverse section through the lining, they appear like narrow lines of condensed chromatin. All nuclei are pointing in one direction and perpendicularly to them are the collagenic fibres of the first layer of connective tissue on which these cells rest. The fibres of the next layer of organized tissue are again perpendicular to the preceding fibres. Thus the number of layers of this dense, fibrous connective tissue can be easily demonstrated in a vertical section through the wall. The individual muscle fibres start to atrophy under the pressure of the growing parasite, but this atrophy is only seldom accompanied by a lymphoid infiltration. Sometimes complete bundles of muscle fibres disappear and the connective tissue layers of the inner perimysium coalesce into wider strips of connective tissue. However, the original structure can be identified on the grounds of some solitary, remaining muscle fibres and mainly on the grounds of the persisting original arrangement of the vessels. These changes in the neighbourhood of the parasite lead to a concentration of connective tissue, which is sometimes erroneously identified as a well developed fibrous encapsulation.

In the perimysial connective tissue the first traces of an inflammatory reaction can be observed, when multiplied plasmatic cells are found perivascularly and when there are also activated and multiplying tissue histiocytes. These can be easily identified in cattle as in rabbits by the fine, plasmatic granulation, which makes it possible to distinguish their cytosplasm, while this is not possible in the sessile fibrocytes between the collagenic fibres, of which only the line-like compressed nucleus is visible.

The first more distinct signs of a commencing tissue reaction can be always found to occur in the wall opposite to the opening of the invaginated canal of the cysticercus on the bladder surface. The nuclei of the marginal cells are swollen, the connective tissue under them is saturated, staining yellow with van Giesson. Also the nuclei of the fibrocytes between the fibrils are more distinct and more numerous. These changes remain restricted to the sector of the wall opposite to the opening of the spiral canal of the parasite. The surface of the whole affected area consists of cells ranging from activated up to independent histiocytic cells, and of single exudative cells of the nature of neutrophils and eosinophilic histiocytes. These superficial layers are saturated with exudate, the complete connective tissue layer of the wall is swollen, its stratified arrangement being retained only on the periphery where it adjoins at the outside the loose granulation tissue.

In the later course of inflammatory changes serous exudate concentrates between the affected area of the wall and the parasite, in which an increase of eosinophilic leukocytes is very marked. In older cysticerci there is sometimes a noticeable aggregation of eosinophilic, necrotic cell exudate in the opening of the entrance canal which is dilated by it. On the surface between the histiocytes there is a considerable amount of a fibrinoid substance, the rim of the histiocytes is high, the cells are arranged in rows and also giant cells appear. The granulation tissue with numerous vessels multiplies on the periphery of the inflammatory rim and its infiltration with lymphoid cells increases. In the granulation tissue there occur foci of phagocytic histiocytes. Thus, the histological picture of the affected area of the wall of the lymphatic space, typical of the tissue reaction of *C. bovis*, is gradually completed, while the other portion of the wall remains unchanged and covered with a cellular lining.

In a fully developed inflammation of the area of the affected wall its surface is formed by a rim of pseudotuberculoid cells infiltrated with eosinophilic leukocytes, which accumulate even in the space between the parasite and the wall. A gradual fibrosis occurs in the deeper layer of the rim; sometimes the amount of mucoid substance increases between the young fibroblasts. On the outer periphery of the inflammatory, activated rim a relatively widespread granulation tissue with numerous vessels is formed. This is greatly infiltrated by lymphoid cells and even the capillaries inside it are filled with lymphocytes leading to the formation of lymphatic follicles with pseudogerminal centres. The granulation tissue on the periphery is changed by fibrosis enclosing atrophic muscle fibres.

Characteristic of *C. bovis* is the development of inflammation in the area of the wall of the original lymphatic space at a time when the parasite is still completely viable, this occurring almost always in the area of the wall facing the opening of the spiral canal. The finding of several of these inflammatory areas of the wall separated from each other is not too frequent, but these areas may originate from the movement of the parasite turning and shifting the opening of the spiral canal toward another part of the wall. The movement of the parasite has been confirmed by relatively frequent findings of small spherical formations on the surface of the inflammatory rim consisting of a mass of exudative cells. The relationship of inflammatory changes to the opening of the spiral canal is mostly very marked. Sometimes, however, inflammatory changes are found even in the neighbourhood of one of the pointed ends of the parasite's bladder. Their localization may perhaps be connected with the original polar placement of the scolex and its opening in the larva before it developed its bladder.

The shifting of the parasite may explain even the structures which are so characteristic of the histological picture of muscle cysticercosis. At the border between the acute inflammatory area and the outer area of the lymphoid granulation tissue we often found in the encapsulating connective tissue foci of a hyaline appearance containing several cells with pycnotic nuclei. Others were normal in structure. The striped foci are bordered on the outside and the inside with typical fibrous connective tissue which they enter directly with their ends. Often we found in them even giant cells with multiple nuclei. We believe these to be the sites where the newly formed granulation tissue of the epitheloid rim succumbed differently to necrobiosis under the direct influence of the parasite. After moving the opening of its spiral canal, the granulation tissue covering these sites continued to mature fibrously in the normal way until it covered the attacked area. The foci situated deeper in the encapsulating tissue are characterized by a coarser, basophilic granulation; with Hale's method they stain distinctly and are strongly metachromatic. In the majority of cases they are calcified. We discovered even a direct metaplasia of the connective tissue in the minute foci of the connective tissue bone in the encapsulating connective tissue. Also parts of the nerves in the connective tissue, passing near to the inflammatory reaction to the parasite, become affected and start to atrophy.

The described changes are fairly distinct particularly when related to the morphology of the cysticerci as indicating the stage of development and age. Therefore, we found the speed of development of the inflammatory reaction to be not always uniform.

Together with the spreading of inflammatory changes over the whole periphery we observed also signs of degeneration of the parasite. The pseudo-epithelial rim, originally bordering the parasite, folds as the parasite shrivels. The space evacuated by the parasite becomes at first occupied by serous, later also by cellular exudate, this being entered even by young fibroblasts. During the scarring of these parts of the cyst the area of the inflammatory rim succumbing to necrosis of the type described above and also calcifying, becomes enclosed by the encapsulating connective tissue and forms in it the same characteristic sites.

The resorption cyst being fibrously encapsulated from the outside, originates actually in the final phase of tissue reaction. Its inside is occupied by the shrivelled parasite and a large amount of cellular exudate consisting of eosinophilic cells. Often both the parasite and the exudate are necrotic, sometimes the necrosis spreads to the resorptive inflammatory rim or even to the fibrous capsule. Macroscopically these cysts are yellow, with condensed contents. Sometimes, the collapsed parasite can be extirpated. The developing tissue reaction leads to the resorption of the parasitic remnants and the exudate and to the formation of scars containing a rich, secondary, lymphoid infiltration sometimes enclosing unresorbed and dystrophically calcified remnants of the parasite.

In a number of cases which, however, were not very frequent in comparison with the total number of cysts examined we observed a different course of tissue reaction. Such cases were noted not only in the heart, but also in the skeletal muscles. There, the histiocytes are activated very early, their mitotic division is very distinct and this not only on the very surface of the lymphatic space, in which the parasite is localized. Throughout the thickness of the wall not only the histiocytes, but also the fibroblasts are greatly activated and start to divide. The larger area of connective tissue in the neighbourhood of the lymphatic space becomes saturated very suddenly with cell exudate, particularly with eosinophilic cells and also the young fibroblasts show sudden signs of maturation. The wide inflammatory rim round the parasite is of a spongy structure, containing great numbers of foamy cells and other inflammatory elements. This strong inflammatory activity is also accompanied by a rich lymphocytic infiltration of the whole focus. Macroscopically, these cysts look both in size and shape like normal cysts at an advanced stage of resorption. The parasite, however, was always found at a very early stage of development, sometimes even in its initial stage, but already showing signs of degeneration or even being necrotic and calcified. The necrotic detritus in its neighbourhood also was calcified. Even dispersed areas of collagenous fibres of the encapsulating connective tissue were metaplastically calcified. These findings suggest a strong tissue reaction to the parasite, impeding its normal development and leading to its sudden dystrophy.


## 4. Importance of morphological studies in the research on cysticercosis

Of primary importance for the evaluation of the tissue reaction in cysticercosis is the possibility of identifying the exact age of the larva. Since such data cannot be obtained experimentally in cysticercosis of man, it is necessary to utilize all knowledge available on the development of C. cellulosae in swine and analogous data about C. bovis, which recently has been largely studied. The period in which the cysticercus attains maturity is important, this being the time when the scolex and suckers have become differentiated to such a degree that in the definitive host the larva can change into an adult cestode. This development is completed by the differentiation of the suckers and the rostellum and the capability of the larva to evaginate its reversed scolex into normal position. According to OSTERTAG (1895) C. cellulosae attains this stage of development at the end of 110 days. But, having reached this stage the cysticercus can still continue to grow for a certain period while retaining its typical appearance and capability of further development. OSTERTAG (1897) studying C. bovis found developed larvae after 112 days, describing also in another paper (OSTERTAG 1895) that he had found larger larvae of the same activity even after 28 weeks. SILVERMAN and HULLAND (1961) mentioned a similar length of time for this larva to attain maturity (three months), MCINTOSH and MILLER (1960) stated 10—12 weeks to be the shortest possible time in which development can be completed. According to the last mentioned authors practically no C. bovis remains infectious after 55 weeks. By contrast DEWHIRST et al. (1963) found viable cysticerci as late as 639 days after the infection. These still exhibited signs of normal activity when their scolices were artificially evaginated. On the basis of the large amount of material examined by URQUHART and BROCKLESBY (1965), 21—30 months may be considered the normal period of longevity of C. bovis unless the cysticercus has been destroyed earlier by a strong tissue reaction. The varied course of tissue reaction and the fact that the influence of this reaction has never been considered in relation to the longevity of C. bovis seems to be the main reason for the divergent results obtained mainly by the artificial infection of calves. On the basis of such experiments LEIKINA et al. (1964) mentioned 11 months as the maximum longevity of the cysticercus, while FROYD (1964) in similar experiments found live cysticerci as late as 30 months after the infection. He drew attention to their dystrophic differences in the experimental animals. VAN DEN HEEVER (1968) drew attention to the importance of the site influencing the longevity of the cysticercus. He found most live cysticerci in the voluntary muscles as late as 36 months after an experimental infection while, at the same time, all cysticerci from the heart were dead.

Similarly *C. cellulosae* can survive in man for a long period, perhaps for several years (HENNER 1940). In some extreme cases it was stated that the cysticercus was known to survive for 15—30 years. Cysticerci in swine, however, can never attain such advanced age because these animals are slaughtered earlier. Therefore, a continued proliferation of the zone of growth of the scolex could not be discover in these intermediate hosts. In cerebral cysticercosis of man we found quite frequently an over-age cysticercus with a scolex growing on a long neck. 30 similar forms of *C. bovis* identified reliably from a total of 500 examined cysticerci, obtained from infected cows and especially from 2—5 year-old bullocks confirmed that this cysticercus also can attain the limits of its life in its intermediate hosts.

The histological criteria applied for the evaluation of the vitality of the parasite, of its dystrophy and autolysis, as described in the relevant chapter, are important, because the dystrophy and necrosis of the parasite are closely related to the character of the tissue reaction. DEWHIRST et al. (1963) drew attention to the fact that viability of *C. bovis* may be ascertained macroscopically from the appearance of the connective tissue capsule, this being fine, translucent and hardly visible in live cysticerci, but thickened and of whitish to yellowish colour in dead ones. According to our observations viable *C. bovis* are not surrounded by a connective tissue capsule, but by an interfascicular connective tissue membrane in the muscle in which they are localized (see for example DEWHIRST et al. 1963).

In our opinion the character of the tissue reaction to *C. bovis* and its gradual development suggests a reaction to the live parasite. Particularly marked is the limitation of tissue reaction to a certain zone opposite the opening of the invaginated canal of the cysticercus this indicating the presence of substances evoking the inflammation and concentrating just in these sites. The noteworthy development of tissue reaction at the site facing the parenchymatous portion of the parasite was observed by MEHLHOSE (1909) who maintained that at the start the inflammation spreading over the whole periphery of the bladder looked like a signet ring in histological sections. These striking characteristics of tissue reaction in muscle cysticercosis were described in the monograph by NIEBERLE and COHRS (1961) who noted also a marked accumulation of the newly formed and lymphoidally infiltrated connective tissue at the pointed poles of the parasitic bladder. This may be due to the fact that the growing parasite distends the bundles of muscle fibres which, however, force by functional pressure the growing bladder into the direction of their course being thus responsible for the elongate shape of the bladder. The slow, but considerable dislocation of the muscle bundles at both ends of the cysticercus predilects these sites as places where the proliferation of the newly formed connective tissue is heaviest. Also HOLZ and PEZENBURK (1957) described the marked development of the encapsulating connective tissue in all these predilection sites calling the slitlike space round the parasite the "pericystäre Lymphraum". They discovered in it frequently an accumulation of eosinophilic leukocytes with staining properties slightly different from those in the granulation tissue. This, evidently, seems to be due to the difference between proper eosinophilic leukocytes and cells designated in our descriptions as eosinophilic histiocytes. Moreover, Holz and Pezenburk found lipoids, granular cholesterol and a small amount of fats with unsaturated bonds of oleic acid on the surface of the cysticercus bladder. They considered the liquid permeating the bordering granulation tissue to be composed of mucoproteids, or possibly glycoproteids.

A description of tissue reaction in calves artificially infected with *C. bovis* was also given by SILVERMAN and HULLAND (1961) who observed reactions varying in strength despite the fact that all animals were infected in the same way. The reaction was different even with two cysticerci located close to each other. In addition they observed a dependence of the mode of development of the cysticerci on the intensity of the host's reaction stating that the stronger the reaction, the less advanced the development of the cysticercus. This is in keeping with our findings of cysts which at first resembled older cysts containing a dead and destroyed parasite, while the examination of their necrotic contents revealed larvae with a not yet developed scolex.

Our findings and also records in the literature indicate that in the bovines *C. bovis* evokes mostly an earlier or later, marked tissue reaction which is characterized by a sudden increase of eosinophilic exudation, this being mostly responsible for the dystrophy of the parasite. This tissue reaction starting at the opening of the invaginated canal of the cysticercus scolex on the bladder surface seems to be an immune response to the antigen produced by the parasite. Later, however, it changes into a strong allergic inflammation causing the death of the parasite. This in its last phase of degeneration and possibly under the influence of enzymatic conditions originating through the presence of exudate in the cyst, often results in the spontaneous evagination of the scolex. This description of the development of tissue reaction contradicts the statement by MEHLHOSE (1909) that bacterial contamination of the cysts in the muscles is mainly responsible for the death of the cysticercus. In some instances, however, evidently when the reaction of the host's tissue is not too strong, even a *C. bovis* can reach the age when its invaginated scolex starts to outgrow and then die only of old age. In animals with a high antibody level a strong tissue reaction sets in immediately after infestation and destroys the larvae even before these can reach their normal stage of development.

In contrast to *C. bovis* there is a minimal tissue reaction to a live *C. cellulosae* as evident from our findings and the data in the literature. NIEBERLE and COHRS (1961) maintained that the finding of a decomposed *C. bovis* is more frequent than that of a *C. cellulosae* and also MEYENBURG (1929) stated in his comprehensive study that an inflammatory reaction to *C. cellulosae* is practically nonexistent. The main development of tissue reaction to a *C. cellulosae* has been noted in most cases only in relation to dying or completely necrotic parasites. The fact that the strongest tissue reaction in cerebral cysticercosis was observed in closest proximity to the highly autolyzed parts of the parasite, was mentioned in the Czech literature by HORÁK, JANATA and JEDLIČKA (1933) who observed it in operation material. The character of this reaction is quite typical; the term leptomeningitis cysticercosa used in the older literature and evaluated by SCHWARZHAUT (1929) designated the complex of changes in the meninges, vessels and the brain tissue. This was confirmed by more recent revisions of the histopathology of cerebral cysticercosis by GURŠTEJN (1947), TRELLES and RAVENS (1953), FISCHER (1955) and TRELLES et al. (1967).

MICHAILOV (1940/41) distinguished on the capsule surrounding the parasite layers of granulation and connective tissue which were differently related to each other in the various observations. Only in decomposed cysticerci did this capsule consist of hyaline connective tissue infiltrated on the outer periphery with lymphoid cells.

Also our findings indicate that the resorptive process may cease even while there are still some remnants of the exudate and of the parasite present. In such instances the hyaline capsule and even the remnants of its contents become calcified and persist in the scar for many years. SHOWRAMMA and BHASKERA RUDDY (1963) maintained that tissue reaction in cases without clinical symptoms is less marked suggesting that clinical symptomatology is evoked mainly by arteritis, by the necrotic material in the focus and the formation of a glial connective tissue scar. This hypothesis may be acceptable, because we also found in our observation no. 1 an increasing meningeal reaction of a noninflammatory type, this increase being certainly correlated with the greater numbers of destroyed parasites. However, the fact should be considered that on postmortem of these five cases without clinical symptoms only viable parasites were found. These generally evoke a relatively weak reaction as mentioned also by NAUCK (1930). Thereby the dystrophy of the cysticerci proceeds so differently that, according to HILLER (1941) simultaneous findings of completely destroyed and calcified parasites together with viable parasites do not necessarily indicate a case of reinfection. Rheumatic pains in muscle cysticercosis as mentioned by FERBER (1865) may originate from an affection of the nerves in the external environment of the parasite as noted also in our observations.

Viable parasites in man may be found only accidentally at the sudden death of the host, while the character of tissue reaction in the early developmental stages of the parasite in the brain has practically never been observed directly. Our findings and also other reports indicate the necessity of presupposing that the cysticercus grows very slowly in the meninges and even in the brain tissue without evoking the slightest inflammatory reaction, but causing only a pressure atrophy in its environment. Should there be a closer metabolic contact between the parasite and its host, a high degree of immunological tolerance is likely to arise. The character of the capsule during the first stages of development may actually be compared with a capsule enclosing an only slightly irritating foreign body similar to that described in our extended experiments with the enclosure by healing of methylmetacrylate implants (ŠLAIS 1958). We found a particularly marked similarity in the capsules formed round the cysticerci in the diaphragm, which contained a minimum of cells and vessels. BEREZANTSEV (1962, 1964) did not agree that there was a similarity in tissue reaction round the larval stages of cestodes to the encapsulation of foreign bodies, but he compared both reactions only in experimental sparganosis, describing the encapsulation in cysticercosis only at its later stage. In a developing inflammatory reaction round the degenerating parasite we found also an increased number of mast cells, likewise observed in the capsule of *Sc. fasciolaris* by COLEMAN and DE SALVA (1963). Noteworthy, however, was the low number of eosinophilic granulocytes; the exudate entering the cyst during the shrivelling of the parasite consisted almost exclusively of neutrophilic leukocytes. This circumstance, very often mentioned in the literature, may perhaps be explained in *C. cellulosae* by the low level of antibody associated with a low incidence of parasites. During the autolysis of the cysticerci this seems to be a local reaction to the products of decomposition being manifested by an increased antibody titre especially in the liquor. KEPSKI et al. (1963) attempted in a model experiment to imitate cerebral cysticercosis by the implantation of *C. cellulosae* into the brain of rabbits and by the embolization of *T. solium* eggs and to trace the formation of specific antibody. Antibody was confirmed in 74% of the experimental animals as early as 3 days after the implantation, although the rabbit is not the normal host of this cysticercus. However, no indisputable proof of their specificity could be obtained.

Of a different nature is the tissue reaction to *C. cellulosae* in a massive cerebral cysticercosis. We found even young stages with a more marked connective tissue capsule in which the tissue reaction to necrotic cysts evoked a massive exudation and infiltration of the connective tissue with eosinophilic leukocytes leading to the necrosis and demarcation of the focus. An increased amount of antibody in the host was to be expected mainly because many parasites, retaining their structure, were calcified without signs of autolysis and resorption.

# Conclusions

The confirmation of the fact that *C. cellulosae* and *C. bovis* with a primary localization in the muscles develop in the lymphatic network of the muscles will greatly change the general concept of these parasites. The relatively large variety of other possible sites in the body in which these parasites may develop has been found to be closely related to this adaptation. While findings of *C. pisiformis* and *C. tenuicollis* outside their typical localization in the abdominal cavity are most exceptional, *C. cellulosae* and *C. bovis* are frequently found elsewhere than in the muscles, this being, in fact typical of *C. cellulosae* in some hosts such as man. This unstable localization in the organs does not suggest a lesser grade of specificity, but is related mainly to the different sites in which the oncospheres in different hosts are arrested. This depends mainly on the anatomy of the blood vessels of the intermediate host and also on the size of the oncospheres, which are smaller in *T. solium* (mean diameter 20 µm) than in *Trh. saginatus* (mean diameter 30 by 25 µm).

All these cysticerci live in fluid. While *C. crassiceps*, *C. pisiformis* and *C. tenuicollis* develop in the serous fluid of the body cavities covered with mesothelial lining, *C. cellulosae* and *C. bovis* adapt themselves more closely to the lymphatic system in the various organs, mainly in the muscles. This is also responsible for morphological changes, underlining the greater importance of their bladder which is protecting the scolex anlage of the cestode. The spacious body cavities facilitate the development of the cysticercus and the growth of its bladder, this being indicated by the well-known phenomenon that the bladder of *C. tenuicollis* grows in conformity to the size of its host, attaining an immense size as demonstrated in the abdominal cavity of an elk. The less spacious conditions in the lymphatic system seem to be responsible for the fact that with *C. cellulosae* and *C. bovis* which both pass during their development through similar stages as the cysticerci from the body cavities, the bladder overgrows the scolex portion in a later phase of development and encloses it as we were able to demonstrate. When the cysticercus increases in volume, its bladder protects it against the pressure of the surrounding tissue, which must be quite high in the muscles. The much larger size, the oval shape and the different morphology of the scolex portion of *C. cellulosae* localized in the subarachnoid cavity and in the brain ventricles show clearly that the shape of *C. cellulosae* and *C. bo-*

*vis* in the muscles, which has been considered to be typical, depends on the environment in which they develop.

Tissue reaction to the cysticerci is indistinct particularly in the early stages of development. Reaction is similar to that against a slightly irritating foreign body (especially *C. cellulosae*) which, sometimes, provokes the organism to form a connective tissue capsule. Also the thin connective tissue capsule of *C. pisiformis* and *C. tenuicollis* and its pedunculate fixation to the omentum and mesenterium seems to be analogous to the capsules surrounding other foreign bodies found in the abdominal cavity. *C. crassiceps* does not attach itself and is only found freely in the ascitic fluid of the abdominal cavity or in the fluid of subcutaneous pseudocysts. Tissue reaction is, naturally, different from that to a decomposing parasite and to one which produces antigen more actively as demonstrated by C. *bovis*.

The elucidation of the histological and histochemical structure of the bladder of the cysticercus as a special organ of this larva made it possible to demonstrate its specific importance for the development of the cysticercus in the organism of its host. We also observed several analogous features between the bladder of the cysticercus and the trophoblast of the mammalian embryo. The striking morphological difference between the bladder and the parenchymatous portion with the scolex of the cysticercus revealing its complicated constitution calls for further studies of its physiology and particularly biochemical studies for an explanation of its metabolism.

The still underrated complicacy of the cysticercus organism and its marked division into a bladder with its specific fluid and a parenchymatous portion with the scolex of the future cestode seems to be responsible for the still unsatisfactory results of immunological investigation of this parasite and for the relatively low specificity of antibody needed particularly for serological diagnosis. The preparation of partial antigens separated on morphological criteria will undoubtedly reveal some interesting facts which may even be used in serological diagnosis of bovine ·cysticercosis and contribute to its eradication and the control of taeniarhynchosis in man.

# Summary

New evidence is given on the morphogenesis, histology and pathogenicity of cysticercus larvae of cestodes, particularly of *C. cellulosae* and *C. bovis*, obtained from 11 observations of cysticercosis of man, from material from muscle cysticercosis of swine and cattle and from comparative material of the larvae *Dithyridium, C. crassiceps, C. pisiformis, C. tenuicollis, Strobilocercus fasciolaris* and *Coenurus cerebralis*.

1.    The parenchymatous portion with the invaginated scolex is enclosed in the bladder cavity of *C. cellulosae* and *C. bovis* by the secondary growth of the bladder induced by the specific localization of these parasites.

2.    The bladder of *C. cellulosae* and *C. bovis* is of a different histological constitution than the scolex portion of these parasites and represents a temporary larval organ.

3.    Even if scolices are not present, a differential diagnosis of *C. cellulosae, C. bovis* and *Coenurus cerebralis* can be made on the grounds of a detailed analysis of the histological structure of the bladder wall of the cysticercus.

4.    The localization of *C. cellulosae* in the brain of man changes its morphology owing to the further possibility of growth. Its appearance is typical of this localization.

5.    In the cysticercus larvae of cestodes, the zone of growth of the cells persists in the region of the invaginated scolex. Its further proliferation gives rise to the special form of cysticercus with an outgrown neck and scolex. This form originates when the cysticercus remains for a long time or indefinitely in its intermediate host. The difference between the outgrowth of the scolex in these forms and the physiological process of evagination of the invaginated cysticercus scolex has been demonstrated.

6.    The racemose form of cerebral cysticercosis originates from the extensive growth of the parasite's bladder during the degeneration of the scolex or when the scolex has not yet been developed. For the first time it has been possible to demonstrate this autonomous growth of the cysticercus bladder.

7.    There are certain analogous feature in the development of the cysticercus larva in the organs of its host and in the development of the mamalian embryo. There is

a clear analogy between the bladder of the cysticercus and the trophoblast, these being adaptive organs of the larva and the embryo facilitating development in other organisms.

8.    The changes in the tissues of the cysticercus during aging, dystrophy and auto-lysis can be traced histologically. The choice of suitable methods ensures the histo-logical identification even of necrotic cysticerci and their remnants in a resorbing and scarring parasitic cyst.

9.    In two cases the remnants of early developmental stages of *C. tenuicollis* could be identified in man and the differential, histological diagnosis of all cysticerci which may be discovered in man was describe. In this connection attention was drawn to the many errors in the diagnosis of cysticercosis found in the literature, because certain artifacts and pseudoparasitic formations were misinterpreted as specific structures.

10.    In our studies of the actual localization of *C. cellulosae* and *C. bovis* in the organs we found evidence that the larvae established in the skeletal muscles and in the heart develop in the lymphatic system and, in cerebral cysticercosis, mainly in the subarachnoid cavity.

11.    With the exception of a massive infestation, *C. cellulosae* affects the surrounding tissue for a considerable length of time only as a slowly growing formation dying mostly of age. Only then does the inflammatory reaction to the decomposition products of the parasite set in, this leading to its resorption and to the scarring of the focus.

12.    In muscle cysticercosis of cattle the tissue starts to react while *C. bovis* is still alive, developing in relationship to the opening of the invaginated scolex. This process is accompanied by a marked exudation of eosinophilic leukocytes, and bears the character of a pseudotuberculoid reaction. A resorptive reaction and scarring start to develop round the necrotic parasite and exudate.

# References

ABASOV KH. D., Regular epidemiological patterns in the formation of taeniarhynchosis foci in Azerbaidzhan SSR and the problems relating to the eradication of this helminthic disease. Med. Parazit. (Mosk.) 34 : 439—444, 1965. (In Russian.)

ACHA N., AGUILAR F. J., Studies on cysticercosis in Central America and Panama. Am. J. trop. Med. Hyg. 13 : 48—53, 1964.

AFSHAR A., Cysticercosis in Iran. Ann. trop. Med. Parasit. 61 : 101—103, 1967.

D'ANDREA F., SMALTINO F., TEDESCHI G., Clinical and radiological considerations on cysticercosis located in the fourth ventricle. Acta neurol. 16 : 612—619, 1964.

ANGULO J. J., ROQUE A. L., A multilocular coenurus of *Multiceps* sp. in *Capromys pilorides* (Say, 1822) Desmarest, 1822. J. Parasit. 34 : 96—100, 1948.

ANISHCHENKO N. A., Development of pathological and morphological changes in experimental cysticercosis of goat and swine infected with *Taenia hydatigena* in connection with the migration, growth and development of the parasite's larvae. Riga 1953. (In Russian.)

ANTONOV A., Über die Art der Kapselbildung bei Hirncysticercose. Virchows Arch. path. Anat. 285 : 485—493, 1932.

ANTONOV I. P., Classification of cysticercosis of the brain (human). Zdravookhr. Beloruss. 12 : 46—48, 1966. (In Russian.)

AVLAVIDOV T., KOVCHAZOV G., Experience in the eradication of taeniasis in the Bulgarian People's Republic. Med. Parazit. (Mosk.) 34 : 572—575, 1965. (In Russian.)

BARTELS E., *Cysticercus fasciolaris*. Zool. Jahrb. Anat. 16 : 511—510, 1902.

BECKER B. J. P., JACOBSON S., Infestation of the human brain with *Coenurus cerebralis*. Report of a fourth case. Lancet 261 : 1202—1204, 1951.

BENEDEN E. VAN, Recherches sur le développement embryonnaire de quelques tenias. Arch. Biol. 2 : 183—210, 1881.

BENNINGHOF A., Lehrbuch der Anatomie des Menschen. Bd. I. Allgemeine Anatomie und Bewegungsapparat. 3. Auflage. J. F. Lehmans Verlag, München—Berlin 1944.

BERBLINGER W., Hypophysitis bei Meningitis basalis cysticercosa. Zbl. allg. Path. path. Anat. 50 : 2—8, 1930.

BEREZANTSEV YU. A., Encapsulation of larval cestode stage in the tissues of the intermediate hosts. Acta vet. Acad. Sci. hung. 12 : 89—98, 1962. (In Russian.)

—, Encapsulation of larvae of parasitic nematodes and cestodes in the tissues of vertebrates as a form of parasite-host relationship. Avtoreferat disertacii. Leningrad 1964. (In Russian.)

BIAGI F. F., BRICENO C. E., Diferencias entre *Cysticercus cellulosae* y *C. racemosus*. Rev. Biol. trop. (S. José) 9 : 141—151, 1961.

—, PINA A. P., Presence of antigens in calcareous corpuscles of cysticercus. Rev. Inst. Med. trop. Sao Paulo 6 : 114—116, 1964.

—, VELEZ G., GUTIERREZ M. L., Destruction of cysticercus in hog-flesh. Pren. méd. mex. 28 : 253—256, 1963.

—, —, —, Destrucción de los cisticercos en la carna de cerda parasitada. Bol. Ofic. sanit. panamer. 58 : 303—307, 1965.

—, —, —, The survival of cysticerci in meat prepared for pork sausage. Rev. méd. mex. 46 : 49—50 1966.

BICKERSTAFF E. R., Cerebral cysticercosis common but unfamiliar manifestations. Brit. med. J. 1 : 1055—1058, 1955.

—, SMALL J. M., WOLF A. L., Cysticercosis of the posterior fossa. Brain 79 : 622—634, 1956.

BOJARSKI Z., WALESZKOWSKI J., Cysticercosis of the brain. Wiad. Parazyt. 9 : 571—578, 1963.

BONNAL G., JOYEUX CH., BOSCH P., Un cas de cénurose humaine du à Multiceps serialis (Ger.). Bull. Soc. Path. exot. 26 : 1060, 1933.

BÖHM K., Untersuchungen über Morphologie, Biologie und Entwicklung der Schweinefinne (Cysticercus cellulosae). Wien. tierärztl. Mschr. 4 : 145—156, 1917.

BOTT A., Über einen durch Knospung sich vermehrenden Cysticercus aus dem Maulwurf. Z. Wiss. Zool. 63 : 115—140, 1898.

BRANDT M., Über Gehirncysticercose beim Menschen. Ärzt. Wschr. 13 : 409—412, 1958.

BRANDT T. VON, MERCADO T. I., NYLEN U. M., SCOTT D. B., Observations on function, composition, and structure of cestode calcareous corpuscles. Exp. Parasit. 9 : 205—214, 1960.

—, NYLEN M. U., SCOTT D. B., MARTIN G. N., Observations on calcareous corpuscles of larval Echinococcus granulosus of various geographic origin. Proc. Soc. exp. Biol. (N. Y.) 120 : 383—385, 1965.

—, —, MARTIN G. N., CHURCHWELL F. K., Composition and crystallization patterns of calcareous corpuscles of cestode grown in different classes of hosts. J. Parasit. 53 : 683—687, 1967.

—, SCOTT D. B., NYLEN M. U., PUGH M. H., Variations in the mineralogical composition of cestode calcareous corpuscles. Exp. Parasit. 16 : 382—391, 1965.

BRAUN M., Cestodes. H. G. BRONNS "Klassen und Ordnungen des Tierreiches" 4. Bd. Vermes. Abt. Ib., Leipzig 1894—1900.

BRICENO C. E., BIAGI F., MARTINEZ B., Cisticercosis observaciones sobre 97 casos de autopsia. Pren. méd. mex. 26 : 193—197, 1961.

BRUMPT E., Précis de parasitologie. 6e édit. Masson, Paris 1948.

—, DUVOIR M. E., SAINTON J., Un cas de cénurose humaine du au Coenurus serialis parasite habituel des lapins et des lièvres. Ann. Parasit. hum. com. 12 : 371—393, 1934.

BULNES L. S., Extraction of a free cysticercus in the vitreous chamber. Considerations and surgical treatment. Gac. méd. Méx. 90 : 715—717, 1960.

CABALLERO C. E. y, A case of human cerebral coenurosis in Mexico. Acta zool. mex. 1 : 1—8, 1956.

CADIGAN F. C. jr., STANTON J. S., PRAYOTH TANTICHAROENYOS, VERACHART CHAICUMPA, The lar gibbon as definitive and intermediate host of Taenia solium. J. Parasit. 53 : 844, 1967.

CAMPBELL W. C., The efficacy of surface-active agents in stimulating the evagination of cysticerci in vitro. J. Parasit. 49 : 81—84, 1963.

—, RICHARDSON T., Stimulation of cysticercus evagination by means of surfactants. J. Parasit. 46 : 490, 1960.

CANELAS H. M., Neurocysticercosis: Incidence, diagnosis, and clinical forms. Arch. Neuro-psiquiat. (S. Paulo) 20 : 1—16, 1962.

CAPRON A., ROSE F., The composition of helminth eggs. II. Acid alcohol-resistance in cestodes. Difference in colorability by the Ziehl stain of the embryophores of Taenia saginata and Taenia solium. Bull. Soc. Pathol. exot. 55 : 765—767, 1963.

CHABASSE Y., GENTHON H., Observations sur la fréquence et les localisations de la cysticercose bovine aux abattoirs d'Angers. Rec. Méd. vét. 138 : 1083—1093, 1962.

Cheng T. C., Provenza D. V., Studies on cellular elements of the mesenchyma and of tissues of *Haematoloechus confusus* Ingles, 1932 (Trematoda). Trans. Amer. Micr. Soc. 79 : 170 — 179, 1960.

Chowdhury A. B., Dasgupta B., Ray H. N., On the nature and structure of the calcareous corpuscles in *Taenia saginata*. Parasitology 52 : 153—157, 1962.

Christiansen M., Die Muskelfinne des Rehes und deren Bandwurm (*Cysticercus* et *Taenia cervi* n. sp. ad interim). Z. Parasitenk. 4 : 75—100, 1932.

Chung H. L., Lee C. U., Cysticercosis cellulosae in man with special reference to involvement of central nervous system. Chin. med. J. 49 : 429—445, 1935.

Coleman E. J., Salva S. J. de, Mass cell response to cestode infection. Proc. Soc. exp. Biol. (N. Y.) 112 : 432—434, 1963.

Collin W. K., Electron microscope studies of the muscle and hook systems of hatched onco-spheres of *Hymenolepis citelli* McLeod, 1933 (Cestoda: Cyclophyllidea). J. Parasit. 54: 74 — 88, 1968.

Correa F M. A., Filho F. F., Forjaz S., Martalli N., Cerebral coenurosis: report of a human case. Rev. Inst. Med. trop. S. Paulo 4 : 38—45, 1962.

Craig Ch. F., Faust E. C., Clinical parasitology. Philadephia 1951.

Crome L., Valentine J. C., Pulmonary nodular granulomatosis caused by inhaled vegetable particles. J. clin. Path. 15 : 21—25, 1962.

Crusz H., The early development of the rostellum of *Cysticercus fasciolaris* Rud. and the chemical nature of its hooks. J. Parasit. 33 : 87—98, 1947.

—, Further studies on the development of *Cysticercus fasciolaris* and *Cysticercus pisiformis*, with special reference to the growth and sclerotization of the rostellar hooks. J. Helminth. 22 : 179—198, 1948.

Daccak M. M., Ulcère et pseudo-ulcère en cysticercose. Arch. Mal. Appar. dig. 51 : 1556—1561, 1962.

Després P., Note complémentaire au problème de la cysticercose bovine en Suisse. Schweiz. Arch. Tierheilk. 104 : 116—119, 1962.

—, Rausch W., Diagnosis and the importance of bovine cysticercosis in Switzerland. Schweiz. Arch. Tierheilk. 103 : 506—518, 1961.

Dewhirst L. W., Cramer J. D., Pistor W. J., Bovine cysticercosis. I. Longevity of cysticerci of *Taenia saginata*. J. Parasit. 49 : 297—300, 1963.

—, —, Sheldon J. J., An analysis of current inspection procedures for detecting bovine cysticer-cosis. J. Amer. vet. med. Ass. 150 : 412—417, 1967.

Dixon H. B. F., Lipscomb F. M., Cysticercosis: An analysis and follow up of 450 cases. Med. Res. Council, Spec. Report Ser. No. 299, London 1961.

Dluhoš M., Schejbal V., Pospíšil L., To the problem of candidoses in childhood. Communica-tion at the 12th Czechoslovak Conference of the Society of Pathologists. Prague 1962. (In Czech.)

Dobrovolskaya - Zaitseva E. A., The lymphatic system of the endocardium in man. Arkh. Anat. Gistol. Embriol. 41 : 76—81, 1961. (In Russian).

Dollfus R. P., Etudes critiques sur les tétrahynques. Substance constituant les crochets. Arch. Musée nat. hist. natur. Paris, série 6, 52—53, 1942.

Duplay J., Bérard - Badier M., Cossa P., Ranque J., A propos d'un cas de cénurose cérébrale. Presse méd. 63 : 625—626, 1955.

Dvořáček Č., Cysticercus in the 3rd ventricle as the cause of sudden death during lumbal punc-ture. Prakt. lék 6 : 112—113, 1949. (In Czech).

Eldon - Dew R., Cysticercosis in humans. S. Afr. J. Sci. 63 : 194—197, 1967.

Fedyay V. V., The structure of connective tissue and of the lymphatic system of the myocardium in man. Arkh. Anat. Gistol. Embriol. 40 : 75—81, 1961. (In Russian.)

FERBER H., Verhalten sich die Blasenwürmer in den Muskeln des Menschen völlig symptomlos? Virchows Arch. path. Anat. 32 : 249—255, 1865.

FERKOVIĆ M., The incidence of cysticercosis of the brain. Liječn. Vjesn. 86 : 463—469, 1964.

FIEBIGER J., Die tierische Parasiten der Haus- und Nutztiere, sowie des Menschen. Berlin—Wien 1936.

FISCHER W., Die parasitären Erkrankungen des zentralen Nervensystems und seiner Hüllen. Henke-Lubarschs Handb. spec. path. Anat. 13 : 372—412, 1955.

FREEMAN R. S., Studies on the biology of *Taenia crassiceps* (Zeder, 1800) Rudolphi, 1810 (Cestoda). Can. J. Zool. 40 : 969—990, 1962.

FROYD G., Cysticercosis and hydatid disease of cattle in Kenya. J. Parasit. 46 : 491—496, 1960.

—, The artificial infection of calves with oncospheres of *Taenia saginata*. Res. Vet. Sci. 2 : 243—247, 1961.

—, Intradermal tests in the diagnosis of bovine cysticercosis. Bull. epizoot. Dis. Afr. 11 : 303—306, 1963.

—, The artificial oral infection of cattle with *Taenia saginata* eggs. Res. Vet. Sci. 5 : 434—440, 1964.

—, The longevity of *Cysticercus bovis* in bovine tissues. Brit. Vet. J. 120 : 205—211, 1964.

—, ROUND M. C., Infection of cattle with *Cysticercus bovis* by the injection of onchospheres. Nature (Lond.) 184 : 1510, 1959.

GALLAGHER I. H. H., Chemical composition of hooks isolated from hydatid scolices. Exp. Parasit. 15 : 110—117, 1964.

—, THREADGOLD L. T., Electron-microscope studies of Fasciola hepatica II. The interrelationship of the parenchyma with other organ systems. Parasitology 57 : 627—632, 1967.

GALLAIS P., PAILLAS C., LUIGI M., DEMARCHI J., DESCHIENS R., Étude anatomo-pathologique d'un kyste parasitaire cérébral observé chez l'homme. Bull. Soc. Path. exot. 48 : 830—832, 1955.

GANTSCHEV N., Electrocoagulation of a *Cysticercus subretinalis*. In: Probleme der Konservativen und operativen Therapie in der Augenheilkunde, Leipzig, 1961. Wiss. Zeit. Karl-Marx-Univ. Leipzig 10 : 734—735, 1961.

GELAZIUS J. B., Calcification of *Hydatigera taeniaeformis* larvae. Tr. Amer. Micr. Soc. 81 : 356—364, 1962.

GEMMELL M. A., Natural and acquired immunity factors inhibiting penetration of some hexacanth embryos through the intestinal barrier. Nature (Lond.) 194 : 701—702, 1962.

—, Immunological responses of the mammalian host against tapeworm infections. II. species specificity of hexacanth embryos protecting rabbits against *Taenia pisiformis*. Immunology 8 : 270—280, 1965.

—, Immunological responses of the mammalian host against tapeworm infections. III. species specificity of hexacanth embryos in protecting sheep against *Taenia ovis*. Immunology 8 : 281—290, 1965.

GIBSON T. E., The identification of *Cysticercus bovis*, with special reference to degenerate cysticerci. Ann. trop. Med. Parasit. 53 : 25—26, 1959.

GLÄSER H., Zur Entwicklungsgeschichte des *Cysticercus longicollis* Rud. Z. wiss. Zool. 92 : 540—561, 1909.

GOLDSCHMID J. M., Two unusual cases of cysticercosis in man in Rhodesia. J. Helminth. 40 : 331—336, 1966.

GOTFRÝD O., LOUBAL L., KOSTELNÍK J., Cysticercosis of the temporal lobe. Rozhl. Chir. 37 : 110—113, 1958. (In Czech).

GÖNNERT R., MEISTER G., STRUFE R., WEBBS G., Biological problems in *Taenia solium* infection. Z. Tropenmed. Parasit. 18 : 76—81, 1967.

GUERRERO F. E., Cerebral cysticercosis: Necropsy findings. Rev. ecuator. Med. Cienc. Biol. III : 142—150, 1965.

GRABER M., THOME M., Bovine cysticercosis in Tchad: Present status, etiology, diagnosis, immunity and therapy of this zoonose (Cestoda, Platyhelminthes). Rev. Élev. 17 : 441—466, 1964.

GURSHTEJN I., Cysticercus from the cerebrum. Moskva 1947. (In Russian.)

HAMMER H., Zur Casuistik der sogenannten freien Cysticerken in den Hirnventrikeln. Prag. med. Wschr. 14 : 243—246, 1889.

HAŠKOVEC K., Case of cerebral cysticercosis. Rev. neurol. psych. 11—12, 1929. (In Czech.)

HEEVER L. W. VAN DEN, On the longevity of Cysticercus bovis in various organs of a bovine. J. Parasit. 53 : 1168, 1968.

HEILMAN P., Beitrag zur Pathologie der Hirncysticercose. Virchows Arch. path. Anat. 286 : 176—182, 1932.

HEINZ H. J., ARON L., Studies on Cysticercus cellulosae. S. Afr. J. med. Sci. 31 : 61—66, 1966.

—, KLINTWORTH G. K., Cysticercosis in the aetiology of epilepsy. S. Afr. J. med. Sci. 30 : 32—36, 1965.

HENNER K., Cysticercosis of the brain. Neurol. psychiat. čs. 2 : 84—86, 1940. (In Czech.)

—, JEDLIČKA V., Case report. Čas. Lék. čes. 59 : 757—758, 1920. (In Czech.)

—, ŠIMEK J., MACEK Z., JIRÁSEK H., ŠIKL H., Cerebral cysticercosis. Čas. Lék. čes. 85 : 361—368, 1946. (In Czech).

HERZOG G., Über einen Rautengrubencysticercus. Ein Beitrag zur Histologie der Ependymveränderungen. Beitr. path. Anat. 56 : 215—230, 1913.

HERTWIG O., Beitrag zur Frage der Entwicklung der Rinderfinne. Z. Fleisch-u. Milchhyg. 1 : 107 — 115, 1891.

HILLER J., Inspection of cysticercus infested meat and consequent taeniasis in man. Prakt. Lék. (Praha) 21 : 257—261, 1941. (In Czech.)

HOLZ J., PEZENBURG E., Histologische und histochemische Untersuchungen an den Hüllen von Cysticercus inermis. Mschr. Tierheilk. 9 : 37—43, 1957.

HONER M. R., Studies on the epidemiology of cysticercosis bovis in the Netherlands. I. The dynamics of cysticercosis bovis. Mededeel. Landbouwhogesch. Wageningen 63 : 1—9, 1963.

HORÁK, JANOTA, JEDLIČKA V., Successful extirpation of a cysticercus from the meninges in the left region of Rolando. Čas. Lék. čes. 38 : 1141—1144, 1933. (In Czech.)

IZQUIERDO L. E., Cerebral cysticercosis. Acta politecn. mex. 2 : 275—284. 1960.

JAKOBSON L., Über Cysticercus cellulosae cerebri et musculorum, mit besonderer Berücksichtigung der den Parasiten einschliessenden Kapselwand. Z. Psychol. Neurol. 21 : 119—136, 1907.

JANICKI C. VON, Über die Embryonalentwicklung von Taenia serrata Goeze. Z. wiss. Zoll. 87 : 685—724, 1907.

JOHRI L. N., A morphological and histochemical study of egg formation in a cyclophyllidean cestode. Parasitology 47 : 21—29, 1957.

JONES A. W., SEGARRA J. M., WYANT K. D., Growth and hatching of taeniid eggs. J. Parasit. 46 : 170—174, 1960.

KAHLDEN V. C., Über Wucherungsvorgänge am Ependymepithel bei Gegenwart von Cysticercen. Beitr. path. Anat. 21 : 297—307, 1897.

KARPÍŠEK J., VALACH V., Cysticercus racemosus in the pia mater with a clinical picture of apoplexy. Čs. Neurol. Psychiat. 15 : 179—183, 1952. (In Czech.)

KEPSKI A., SZLAMINSKI Z., ZAPART W., Serological tests in experimental cerebral cysticercosis in rabbits. Acta parasit. polon. 11 : 133—143, 1963.

KHELIMSKIY A. M., Cysticercosis of the brain, heart and skeletal muscles. Med. Parazit. (Mosk.) 31 : 610—611, 1943. (In Russian.)

Kitaoka T., Cerebral cysticercosis; Report of a surgically treated case. Hiroshima J. med. Sci. 39—45, 1962.

Kleibel A., Observations on the occurrence of *Cysticercus bovis* in St. Pölten abattoir. Wien. tierärztl. Mschr. 48 : 469—469, 1961.

Klika E., Meninges of man and higher mammals. Babákova sb., sv. 11, Praha 1959. (In Czech.)

Kocher R., Die pathologisch-anatomischen Veränderungen des Gehirns bei Cysticercus racemosus. Beitr. path. Anat. 50 : 338—360, 1911.

Kosminkov N. E., Diagnosis of cysticercosis of cattle with the allergical method. Doklady VASNIL No. 1 : 32—34, 1965. (In Russian.)

—, Filippov V. V., The use of polystirol latex in the live diagnosis of cysticercosis in cattle. Doklady VASNIL No. 5 : 37—38, 1967. (In Russian.)

Koudela K., Rinderfinnigkeit und Geschlecht der befallenen Tiere. Die Fleischwirtschaft 46 : 1233—1234, 1966.

—, The dynamism of *Cysticercus bovis* regression in spontaneously invaded cattle. Acta Univer. Agric. 15 : 81—85, 1967.

Kovalev N. E., Survival rate of *Cysticercus bovis* in different culinary methods of preparing Cysticercus-infested beef. Med. Parazit. (Mosk.) 34 : 566—570, 1965. (In Russian.)

Kozma M., Gellért A., from Rényi - Vámos F., Das innere Lymphgefässystem der Organe. Budapest 1960.

Kratter J., Böhmig L., Ein freier Gehirncysticercus als Ursache plötzlichen Todes. Beitr. path. Anat. 21 : 25—42, 1897.

Kufs H., Multiple Cysticerken im Gehirn und Entwicklung von unbefruchteten Bandwurmeiern in den Cysticerkenmembranen. Arch. Psychiat. Nervenkr. 186 : 361—370, 1951.

—, Die Entstehung unbefruchteter Bandwurmeier in den Finnenmembranen, ein neues entwicklungsdynamisches Phänomen, bewiesen an *Cysticercus cellulosae, Cysticercus bovis* und *Echinococcus cysticus*. Virchows Arch. path. Anat. 322 : 73—84, 1952.

Kunsemüller F., Zur Kenntnis der polycephalen Blasenwürmer. Zool. Jahrb. Anat. 18 : 507—538, 1903.

Lafon R., Gros C., Labange R., Vlatovitch B., Libstein M., Concerning three cases of neural cysticercosis. Rev. Neurol. 96 : 9—18, 1957.

Larsh J. E., Race G., Esch G. W., A histopathological study of mice infected with the larval stage of *Multiceps serialis*. J. Parasit. 51 : 45—52, 1965.

Lee D. L., The structure and composition of the helminth cuticle. Advanc. Parasit. 4 : 187—254, 1966.

Lee H. H. K., Jones A. W., Wyant K. D., Development of the taeniid embryophore. Tr. Amer. Micr. Soc. 78 : 355—357, 1959.

Leikina E. S., Moskvin S. N., Sokolovskaya O. M., Poletaeva O. G., The longevity of *Cysticercus bovis* and development of immunity in cysticercosis. Med. Parazit. (Mosk.) 6 : 694 to 700, 1964. (In Russian.)

Leuckart R., Die menschlichen Parasiten und die von ihnen herrührenden Krankheiten. I. Band. Leipzig u. Heidelberg. 1863.

—, Die Parasiten des Menschen und die von ihnen herrührenden Krankheiten. I. Band, I. Abt., 2. Aufl., Leipzig u. Heidelberg, 1879—1886.

Lipschitz R., Hefer A. G., Schmaman A., Early manifestation of cerebral tapeworm cyst disease — a case report. S. Afr. Med. J. 42 : 34—5, 1967.

Logachev E. D., The tissue character and the physiological significance of subcuticular cells in cestodes. Dokl. AN SSSR 77 : 161—163, 1951. (In Russian.)

—, The thin structure of the surface cuticle in trematodes and cestodes. Dokl. AN SSSR 103 : 941—943, 1955. (In Russian.)

—, Contribution to the morphology of the connective tissue of larval forms of cestodes. Rab. gelm. k 80-letiyu akad. K. I. Skrjabina, pp. 206—208, Moskva 1958. (In Russian.)

—, The structure and nature of the tissue of cuticular coverings in cysticerci. Dokl. AN SSSR 125 : 1390—1392, 1959. (In Russian.)

—, The tissue character of the submerged epithelium of cestodes. Tr. inst. zool. 11 : 137—139, 1960. (In Russian.)

—, Luminescent-microscope investigations of cuticular structures in helminth larvae. Tezisy dokl. nauch. konf. Vsevojuzn. obshch. gelm., Part 2, pp. 102—103, 1962. (In Russian).

—, New description of the cell nuclei of the connective tissue and of the sexual chromatin of the somatic cells in *Fasciola hepatica*. Dokl. Nauch. konf. posv. pervomu vypusku vrachej Kemerovskogo med. inst., Kemerovo 45—48, 1962. (In Russian.)

—, Micromorphological investigations of the bladder wall of two *Coenurus* species. Materialy k nauch. konf. Vsesoyuzn. obshch. gelm., Part 1, Moskva 1964. (In Russian.)

LOMBADRO L., MATEOS J. H., Cerebral cysticercosis in Mexico. Neurology (Minneap.) 11 : 824—828, 1961.

LOPEZ F., ESCANDON A., Cysticercosis of the central nervous system. Clinical and pathological study of 58 cases. Antioquia med. 14 : 729—743, 1965.

LUCKER J. T., VEGORS H. H., Vaccination against beef measles. J. Anim. Sci. 284, 1965.

LUMSDEN R. D., Cytological studies on the absorptive surfaces of cestodes. II. The synthesis and intracellular transport of protein in the strobilar integument of *Hymenolepis diminuta*. Z. Parasitenk. 28 : 1—13, 1966.

—, Cytological studies on the absorptive surfaces of cestodes. I. The fine structure of the strobilar integument. Z. Parasitenk. 27 : 355—382, 1966.

—, BYRAM J., The ultrastructure of cestode muscle (*Calliobothrium verticillatum, Phyllobothrium foliatum, Lacistorhychus tenuis, Hymenolepis diminuta*). J. Parasit. 53 : 326—342, 1967.

MACHNICKA - ROGUSKA B., Preparation of *Taenia saginata* antigens and chemical analysis of antigenic fractions. Acta parasit. pol. 13 : 337—347, 1965.

—, ZWIERZ C., Haemagglutination reaction in people with *Taenia saginata* invasion. Wiad. Parazyt. 10 : 467—468, 1964. (In Polish.)

—, —, Serological studies on *Taenia saginata*. Acta parasit. pol. 14 : 27—33, 1966.

MAGDIEV R. R., DZHABRIEV N. I., ABUNAGIMOV KH. Z., ZUEVA E. V., ARUTYUNOVA A. A., EMYASHEVA Z. I., STRELNIKOVA G. A., Organization of measures for the control of taenia-rhynchosis for the purpose of its eradication. Med. Parazit. (Mosk.) 34 : 133—139, 1965. (In Russian.)

MARGOLENA L. A., Ziehl - Neelsen's stain for skin sections to show wool and hair follicles. Stain Technol. 38 : 145—148, 1963.

MARÍN G., HERNÁNDEZ TAYAS H. H., GONZÁLES E. F., BOUZAS F. A., AGÜERO BELLO, Cerebral cysticercosis. A report of 2 autochthonous cases. Rev. cuba. Trop. 19 : 63—73, 1967.

MARSCHAND F., Ein Fall von sogenannten *Cysticercus racemosus* des Gehirns. Virchows Arch. path. Anat. 75 : 104—112, 1879.

MARTINEZ G., GIULIANI B., Singolare caso si broncopolmonite de cisticercoidosi. Arch. De Vecchi Anat. pat. 29 : 669—667, 1959.

MAZZOTTI L., The use of ultraviolet light as a help to ease the detection of *Cysticercus cellulosae*. Rev. Invest. Salud públ. 26 : 90—91, 1966.

—, DAVALOS A., MARTINEZ - MARANON R., Natural and experimental infection of different mammal species by *Cysticercus cellulosae*. Rev. Inst. Salubr. Enferm. trop. (Méx) 25 : 151—162, 1965.

MCINTOSH A., MILLER D., Bovine cysticercosis, with special reference to the early development stages of *Taenia saginata*. Amer. J. vet. Res. 21 : 69—177, 1960.

MEHLHOSE R., Über das Vorkommen von Bakterien in den Echinokokken und Cysticerken und ihre Bedeutung für das Absterben dieser Zooparasiten. Zbl. Bakt., I Abt. Orig. 52 : 43—74, 1909.

MENNICKE L., Über zwei Fälle von *Cysticercus racemosus*. Beitr. path. Anat. 21 : 243—263, 1897.

MÉRA A., ANDRÁSOFSZKY A., WAITSUK P., GYERGYAY F., Cysticercosis of the brain assuming an appearance of increased intracranial pressure. Rum. med. Rev. 5 : 54—58, 1961.

MEYENBURG H. VON, Die quergestreifte Muskulatur. Henke-Lubarsch, Handbuch der speziellen pathologischen Anatomie und Histologie, 9. Band, 1. Teil, J. Springer, Berlin 1923.

MONIEZ R., Essay monographique sur les cysticerques. Travaux Inst. Zool. Lille, Station Maritime Wimereux, Paris 3 : 1—190, 1880.

MIKHAILOV G., Cysticercosis in man from sectioned material of the department. Godichnik univ. K. Ochridski, Sofia 20 : 382—393, 1940/41. (In Bulgarian.)

MONNÉ L., On the external cuticles of various helminths and their role in the host-parasite relationship. A histochemical study. Ark. Zool. 12 : 343—358, 1959.

—, On the physiological role of the polyphenols in cell and tissue envelopes. Ark. Zool 13 : 287 — 298, 1960.

MORSETH D. J., Ultrastructure of developing taeniid embryophores and associated structures. Exp. Parasit. 16 : 207—217, 1965.

—, Chemical composition of embryophoric block of *Taenia hydatigena*, *Taenia ovis* and *Taenia pisiformis* eggs. Exp. Parasit. 18 : 347—354, 1966.

—, The fine structure of the tegument of adult *Echinococcus granulosus*, *Taenia hydatigena* and *Taenia pisiformis*. J. Parasit. 52 : 1074—1085, 1966.

—, Observations on the fine structure of the nervous system of *Echinococcus granulosus*. J. Parasit. 53 : 492—500, 1967.

NAUCK E. G., Gehirncystizerkosis. Arch. Schiffs- und Tropenhyg. 34 : 158—161, 1930.

NIEBERLE - COHRS P., Lehrbuch der speziellen pathologischen Anatomie der Haustiere 4. Aufl. VEB G. Fischer Verlag, Jena 1961.

ODAMTTEN S. E., LAING W. N., Cysticercosis of the brain. (Memoranda). Ghana Med. J. 6 : 97 — 105, 1967.

D'OLIVEIRA C. G., Cysticercosis with localization in skeletal muscle. A report of 2 cases. Med. Bull. Stand. Oil Co. 27 : 245—57, 1967.

ORIHARA M., Studies on *Cysticercus fasciolaris*, especially on differences of susceptibility among uniform strains of the mouse. Jap. J. Vet. Res. 10 : 37—56, 1962.

OSTERTAG R., Handbuch der Fleischbeschau. II. Edit. Stuttgart 1895.

—, Beitrag zur Frage der Entwicklung der Rindenfinne und der Selbst-Heilung der Rindenfinnenkrankheit. Z. Fleisch- u. Milchhyg. 8 : 1—5, 1897.

—, Handbuch der Fleischbeschau. Band II, 6. Aufl., Stuttgart 1913.

PAVLOVA L. I., Morphological and histochemical investigation of the structure of eggs in *Taeniarhynchus saginatus* (Goeze, 1782). Helminthologia 6 : 125—133, 1965a. (In Russian.)

—, Cytological investigation of the development of female genital organs in *Taeniarhynchus saginatus* (Goeze, 1782). Helminthologia 6 : 135—144, 1965b. (In Russian.)

PAWLOWSKI Z., Statistical analysis of 1,200 cases of taeniarhynchosis observed in the years 1953—1962. Wiad. Parazyt. 10 : 395—400, 1964. (In Polish.)

PENCE D. B., The fine structure and histochemistry of the infective eggs of *Dipylidium caninum*. J. Parasit. 53 : 1041—154, 1967.

PETROVICKÝ O., Generalized cysticercosis accompanied by a toxoplasma infection. Čs. parasit. 3 : 77—80, 1956. (In Czech.)

PETRŮ M., VOJTĚCHOVSKÁ M., Incidence of taeniarhynchosis in Prague and surroundings. Čs. Parasit. 10 : 273—276, 1963. (In Czech.)

—, —, Syrovátka A., Some factors contributing to the further spreading of *Taeniarhynchus saginatus*. Prakt. Lék. 46 : 379—381, 1966. (In Czech.)

Piazza M., Gaddo M. di, Sulla cisticercosi umana. Pathologica 54 : 809—810, 1962.

Pintner T., Studien über Tetrahynen II. Mitteilung. Über eine Tetrahynenlarve aus dem Magen von Heptanchus, nebst Bemerkungen über das Excretionssystem verschiedener Cestoden. S.-B. Akad. Wiss. Wien, math.—nat. Kl. 105 : 652—682, 1896.

Pita R. V. de, Velez - Pratt G. V., Biagi F. F., Immunofluorescence detectable antigens in calcareous corpuscles of *Cysticercus cellulosae*. Rev. Fac. Med. Univ. Méx. 7 : 379—383, 1965.

Potselueva V. A., Development of *Cysticercus pisiformis* in the organism of the rabbit. Rab. gelm. pp. 564—566, Moskva 1953. (In Russian).

Powell S. J., Proctor E. M., Wilmot A. J., MacLeod I. N., Cysticercosis and epilepsy in Africans: A clinical and serological study. Ann. Trop. Med. Parasit. 60 : 152—158, 1966.

—, —, —, Barnett A. M., Neurological complication of cysticercosis in Africans: A clinical and serological study. Ann. Trop. Med. Parasit. 60 : 159—164, 1966.

Price E. W., A note on hepatic cysticercosis, with the proposal of a new variety of *Taenia saginata*. J. Alabama Acad. Sci. 32 : 257—261, 1961.

Proctor E. M., Powell S. J., Elsdon - Dew R., The serological diagnosis of cysticercosis. Ann. trop. Med. Parasit. 60 : 146—151, 196.

Przeorska B., A case of cysticercosis of the eye in a boy. Wiad. Parazyt. 13 : 705—6, 1967.

Rabl R., Chronische Meningitis bei Cysticercus. Zbl. allg. Path. path. Anat. 98 : 408—421, 1958.

Race G. J., Larsh J. E., Esch G. W., Martin J. H., A study of the larval stage of *Multiceps serialis* by electron microscopy. J. Parasit. 51 : 364—369, 1965.

—, Martin J. H., Larsh J. E., Esch G. W., A study of the adult stage of *Taenia multiceps* (*Multiceps serialis*) by electron microscopy. J. Elisha Mitschell Scientific Soc. 82 : 44—57, 1966.

Recklinghausen von, Das Lymphgefässsystem. Strickers Handbuch der Lehre von den Geweben des Menschen und der Tiere. I. : 214—250, 1871.

Rehnová M., Results of investigations into the infestation of rural populations with *Taeniarhynchus saginatus*. Prakt. Lék. 47 : 605, 1967. (In Czech.)

Robinson R. G., Coenurosis of the central nervous system. Wld. Neurol. 3 : 35—42, 1962.

Roger H., Sautet J., Paillas J. E., Un cas de cénurose de la fosse cérébrale postérieure. Rev. neurol. 74 : 319—321, 1942.

Rössler P., Über den feineren Bau der Cysticerken. Zool. Zbl. 16 : 423—448, 1902.

Rothman A. H., Electron microscopy studies of tapeworms. Trans. Amer. Micr. Soc. 82 : 22—30, 1963.

—, Ultrastructural studies of enzyme activity in the cestode cuticle. Exp. Parasit. 19 : 332—338, 1966.

—, Lee D. L., Histochemical demonstration of dehydrogenase activity in the cuticle of cestodes. Exp. Parasit. 14 : 333—336, 1963.

Rybická K., Embryogenesis in cestodes. Advanc. Parasit. 4 : 107—186, 1966.

Round M. C., Observation on the possible role of filth flies in the epizootiology of bovine cysticercosis in Kenya. J. Hyg. (London) 59 : 505—513, 1961.

Rycke P. H. de, Scolex of *Cysticercus fasciolaris*. Nature (Lond.) 198 : 1110—1111, 1963.

—, Grembergen G. van, Etude sur l'évagination de scolex d'*Echinococcus granulosus*. Z. Parasitenk. 25 : 518—525, 1965.

—, —, Study on the evagination of *Cysticercus pisiformis*. Z. Parasitenk. 27 : 341—349, 1966.

Saint - Remy G., Le développement embryonnaire de *Taenia serrata* Goeze. Arch. Parasit. 4 : 143—156, 1901.

Salganik E., Cerebral cysticercosis. Izd. "Kartya Moldovenyaske" Kishinev 1967. (In Russian.)

SAMSONOV V. A., MESHKOVA A. N., Generalized form of cysticercosis with an extensive infestation of the cerebrum, the skin and the skeletal muscles. Arkh. patol. 29 : 73—77, 1967. (In Russian.)

SAPUNAR J., MORALES E., A case of cerebral cysticercosis. Bol. Chil. Parasit. 18 : 16—19, 1963.

SCHAAF H., Zur Kenntnis der Kopfanlage der Cysticerken, insbesondere des Cysticerkus *Taeniae solii*. Zool. Jahrb. Anat. 22 : 435—476, 1905.

SCHILLER E. L., The histogenesis of cuticle with cestode genus *Taenia*. J. Parasit. 46 : 9—10, 1960.

SCHMIDT - HOENSDORF F., PEZENBURG E., Die Entstehung unbefruchteter Bandwurmeier in den Finnenmembranen. Eine Erwiderung. Virchows Arch. path. Anat. 331 : 623—625, 1958.

SCHÖPPLER H., Über einen Fall von *Cysticercus cellulosae* im 4. Ventrikel als plötzliche Todesursache. Zbl. allg. Path. path. Anat. 17 : 945—951, 1906.

SCHWARZHAUPT W., Über Cysticerken im Gehirn. Inaugural — Dissertation, Köln am Rhen 1929.

SCOTT D. B., NYLEN M. U., BRAND v. T., PUGH M. H., The mineralogical composition of the calcareous corpuscles of *Taenia taeniaeformis*. Exp. Parasit. 12 : 445—458, 1962.

SHOWRAMMA A., REDDY B. D., Silent cysticercosis of the brain. An analysis of five cases with special reference to histopathology. Indian J. Path. Bact. 6 : 142—147, 1963.

SHULMAN E. S., KAMINSKIY M. I., Ways of eradicating infections caused by *Taenia* (formerly *Taeniarhynchus*) tapeworms in the Ukraine. Problems of medical parasitology and the prevention of infection. pp. 510—517, Moscow 1964. (In Russian.)

SIDDIQUE E. H., The cuticle of cysticerci of *Taenia saginata*, *T. hydatigena* and *T. pisiformis*. Quar. J. Micr. Sci. 104 : 141—144, 1963.

SIGMUND A., The dissemination of muscle cysticercosis. Čas. Lék. čes. 66 : 1244—1247, 1927. (In Czech.)

SILVERMAN P. H., Studies on the biology of some tapeworms of the genus *Taenia*. I. Factors affecting hatching and activation of taeniid ova and some criteria of their viability. Ann. trop. Med. Parasit. 48 : 207—215, 1954a.

—, Studies on the biology of some tapeworms of the genus *Taenia* II. The morphology and development of the taeniid hexacanth embryo and its enclosing membranes, with some notes on the state of development and propagation of gravid segments. Ann. trop. Med. Parasit. 48 : 356—366, 1954b.

—, HULLAND T. J., Histological observations on bovine cysticercosis. Res. Vet. Sci. 2 : 248—252, 1961.

SKVORTZOV A. A., Egg structure of *Taeniarhynchus saginatus* and its control. Zool. Zhurnal 21 : 10—18, 1942. (In Russian.)

SMYTH J. D., The biology of cestode life cycles. Techn. Com. Commonwealth Bureau of Helmint. No. 34, St. Albans, Herts, England, 1963.

—, Observations on the scolex of *Echinococcus granulosus*, with special reference to the occurrence and cytochemistry of secretory cells in the rostellum. Parasitology 54 : 515—526, 1964.

—, Studies on tapeworms physiology. XI. In vitro cultivation of *Echinococcus granulosus* from protoscolex to the strobilate stage. Parasitology 57 : 111—133, 1967.

—, CLEGG J. A., Egg-shell formation in trematodes and cestodes. Exp. Parasit. 8 : 286—323, 1959.

—, HOWKINS A. B., BARTON M., Factors controlling the differentiation of the hydatid organism, *Echinococcus granulosus*, into cystic or strobilar stages in vitro. Nature, London 211 : 1374—1377, 1966.

SOKOLOVSKAYA O. M., MOSKVIN S. N., Agglutination test with latex as a method of vital diagnosis of cysticercosis of cattle. Med. Parazit. (Mosk.) 36 : 138—143, 1967. (In Russian.)

SPINA - FRANCA A., Cisticercose do sistema nervoso central. Rev. paul. Med. 48 : 59—70, 1956.

—, Síndrome liquórica da neurocysticercose. Arch. Neuro-psiquiat. (S. Paulo) 19 : 307—314, 1961.

—, Aspectos biológicos da neurocysticercose: Alterações do líquido cefalorraquidiano. Arch. Neuro-psiquiat. (S. Paulo) 20 : 17—30, 1962.

STEFANKO S., ŻEBROWSKI S., The morphology of cerebral paragonimiasis. Acta med. pol. 2 : 111 — 122, 1961.

STĘPIEN Z., Cysticercosis in Poland. J. Neurosurg. 6 : 505—513, 1962.

STUCHLÍK J., Cerebral cysticercosis — case reports. Čas. Lék čes. 67 : 1736, 1928. (In Czech.)

ŠLAIS J., Histologischer Nachweis von Parasiten in nekrotischen und verkalkten Gebilden (Linguatula, Cysticercus). Zbl. allg. Path. path. Anat. 101 : 200—207, 1960.

—, Late tissue reaction in cerebral cysticercosis of man. Výhled (semináře pro doškolování veter. lékařů v Pardubicích) I/VI: 19, 1962. (In Czech.)

—, Zur Pathogenese der Oxyurengranulome. Zbl. allg. Path. path. Anat. 103 : 214—222, 1962.

—, A threadworm granuloma in the human liver. Helminthologia 4 : 479—484, 1962/63.

—, Histological demonstration of dead linguatula larvae in the liver of man. Čs. parasit. 10 : 163 — 169, 1963. (In Czech.)

—, Histochemistry of tissue resorption of experimentally implanted pinworms. Čs. parasit. 11 : 263—272, 1964.

—, Histologischer Nachweis der Reste von Echinococcuscysten. Čs. Parasit. 11 : 339—341, 1964.

—, Histologic studies in cysticercosis of the brain. Wiad. Parazyt. 10 : 313—314, 1964.

—, Demonstration of the parasite and tissue reaction in cerebral cysticercosis. Čs. Parasit. 12 : 263—297, 1965. (In Czech.)

—, Morphology of the agent of cerebral cysticercosis. Čs. Pat. 1 : 65—76, 1965. (In Czech.)

—, Befunde von frühen Entwicklungsstadien des Cysticercus in der Leber des Menschen. Zbl. allg. Path. path. Anat. 108 : 316—321, 1965.

—, Zur Morphologie und Entstehung der invaginierten Cysticerken mit einem herausgewachsenen Skolex. Z. Parasitenk. 27 : 25—42, 1966.

—, Beitrag zur Morphogenese des Cysticercus cellulosae und C. bovis. Folia parasit. (Praha) 13 : 73—92, 1966.

—, Die Analogie zwischen dem Trophoblast und dem Bläschen der Cysticercuslarven der Bandwürmer. Anat. Anz. 118 : 495—502, 1966.

—, The functional histology of the bladder wall of some cysticerci. Folia parasit. (Praha) 13 : 193 — 204, 1966.

—, The importance of the bladder for the development of the cysticercus. Parasitology 56 : 707 — 713, 1966.

—, The morphology of Cysticercus racemosus and the determination of the cysticercus species. Folia parasit. (Praha) 14 : 27—34, 1967.

—, The location of the parasites in muscle cysticercosis. Folia parasit. (Praha) 14 : 217—224, 1967.

—, Die Morphologie und histologische Diagnostik des Parasiten bei der Gehirncysticerkose. Acta neuropath. (Berl.) 10 : 295—307, 1968.

—, KALUŠ M., Racemose form of cerebral cysticercosis. Čs. Pat. 3 : 80—87, 1967. (In Czech.)

THREADGOLD L. T., An electron-microscope study of the tegument and associated structures of Dipylidium caninum. Quar. J. micr. Sci. 103 : 135—140, 1962.

—, An electron microscope study of the tegument and associated structures of Proteocephalus pollanicoli. Parasitology 55 : 467—472, 1965.

TOMIYASU U., RAMSEYER J. C., BAKER R. N., Wernicke-like syndrome with chronic meningitis: A clinical neuropathological study of a patient with cysticercosis. Bull. Los Angeles neurol. Soc. 31 : 72—83, 1966.

TRELLES J. O., Cerebral cysticercosis. Wld Neurol. 2 : 488—497, 1961.

—, PALOMINO L., CACERES A., Histopathology of the cerebral cysticercosis. Acta neuropath. (Berl.) 8 : 115—132, 1967.

—, Ravens R., Estudios sobre neurocisticercosis. II. Lesiones vasculares, meningeas, ependimarias y neurológicas. Rev. Neuropsiquiat. (Lima) 16 : 241—271, 1953.

—, Rocca E., Ravens R., Estudios sobre neurocysticercosis I. Sobre la fina estructura de la membrana vesicular quistica y racemosa. — Deducciones patológicas. Rev. Neuro-psiquiat. (Lima) 15 : 1—35, 1952.

Urquhart G. M., Epizootiological and experimental studies on bovine cysticercosis in East Africa. J. Parasit. 47 : 857—869, 1961.

—, Parenteral production of cysticercosis (Cestoda, Mammalia, Host, Diptera, Vector). J. Parasit. 51 : 544, 1965.

—, Brocklesby D. W., Longevity of *Cysticercus bovis*. J. Parasit. 51 : 349, 1965.

Varleta J., Oberhouser E., Weinstein V., Contributions to our knowledge of the chemical pathology of neurocysticercosis. Bol. Chil. Parasit. 16 : 62—66, 1961.

Verster A., Redescription of *Taenia solium* Linnaeus, 1753 and *Taenia saginata* Goeze, 1782. Z. Parasitenk. 29 : 313—328, 1967.

Vidvarthi S. C., Diffuse milliary granulomatosis of the lungs due to aspirated vegetable cells. Arch. Path. 83 : 215—218, 1967.

Virchow R., Helminthologische Notizen. Virchows Arch. path. Annat. 11 : 79—86, 1857.

—, Helmintologische Notizen. 5. Traubenhydatiden der weichen Hirnhaut. Virchows Arch. path. Anat. 18 : 528—535, 1860.

Voge M., Obervations on the structure of the cysticercus of *Taenia hydatigena* Pallas, 1766. Proc. Helm. Soc. Wash. 38 : 62—66, 1962.

—, Observations on the structure of cysticerci of *Taenia solium* and *Taenia saginata* (Cestoda: Taeniidae). J. Parasit. 49 : 85—90, 1963.

Wainwright J., *Coenurus cerebralis* and racemose cyst of the brain. J. Path. Bact. 73 : 347—354, 1957.

Waitz J. A., Studies of the ultrastructure of larval *Hydatigera taeniaeformis*. J. Parasit. 47 (Suppl.): 27, 1961.

—, Histochemical studies of the cestode *Hydatigera taeniaeformis* Batsch, 1786. J. Parasit. 49 : 73—80, 1963.

Watson K. C., Laurie W., Cerebral coenuriasis in man. Lancet 269 : 1321—1322, 1955.

Webbe G., The hatching and activation of taeniid ova in relation to the development of cysticercosis in man. Z. Tropenmed. Parasit. 18 : 354—69, 1967.

Weiser F., Zur Differentialdiagnose der parasitären Lungenerkrankungen—Cysticercose—Pentostomiasis. Beitr. Klin. Tuberk. 98 : 239—254, 1942.

Zenker F. A., Über den *Cysticercus racemosus* des Gehirns. Beiträge zur Anatomie und Embryologie als Festgabe für Jakob Henle, pp. 119—140, 1882.

Zhdanov D. A., General anatomy and physiology of the lymphatic system. Leningrad 1952. (In Russian.)

# Acknowledgments

In publishing this book it is pleasure to thank Professor Dr. J. Vaněk from Plzeň for his invaluable assistance and support of my studies on cerebral cysticercosis. I am also greatly indebted to Professor Dr. B. Bednář and to Professor Dr. V. Jedlička from Prague for providing more important material for my studies. I wish to express my sincerest thanks to Academician O. Jírovec and to Professor Dr. B. Rosický for their critical evaluation of all parasitological problems. The valuable comments on the egg and oncosphere of taeniids, made by Dr. K. Rybicka from Warsaw, are highly appreciated. I am most grateful to Professor Dr. S. B. Kendall from Weybridge not only for his general critical comments on the manuscript but for his invaluable help in revising the difficult translation of the manuscript into English provided by Mrs. E. Kalinová. I am indebted to Dr. D. Hulínská for her assistance in the study on the structure of the cysticercus bladder and Mrs. V. Žákavcová and Mrs. M. Somolová for their technical assistance in the histological elaboration of the material.

# Explanation of the plates

## Plate I

Fig. 1. Section through a young *C. cellulosae* in a cavity in the brain tissue. The bladder starts to grow round the parenchymatous portion. Fig. 2. Section through a *C. cellulosae* with its bladder almost enclosing the parenchymatous portion. Haematoxylin-eosin (28×).

## Plate II

Fig. 1 and 2. Histological section through the opening of the spiral canal in two *C. bovis*. Their parenchymatous portion is not yet completely recessed in the bladder cavity. The cuticle of the spiral canal constitutes also the surface round the opening and passes into the surface of the bladders.The parenchyma is packed with calcareous corpuscles. Weigert-van Gieson (Fig. 1 40×, Fig. 2 24×). Fig. 3. Histological section through the opening and through part of the entrance canal in *C. bovis*. The tissue is of the same composition as that of the bladder wall, without calcareous corpuscles. The lining of the canal consists only of the hypertrophic cuticle of the bladder surface. Goldner (30×).

## Plate III

Fig. 1. Bladder wall of *C. cellulosae* from the muscles of swine in expanded position showing the dilated branches of the duct system and the wartlike surface of the cuticle. On the base of the protuberances are the contracted subcuticular muscle groups(a), which are followed by a layer of subcuticular cells(b), and some fibres(f) of the main muscles of the wall. In the wall are sections of the ducts of the upper(c) and the lower(d) network and the ducts(h) which connect both systems. Fig. 2. Shrunken wall of the same *C. cellulosae*. The strands of contracted subcuticular muscle groups are clearly visible at the base of the wartlike formations. The subcuticular cells are still arranged in a row. Haematoxylin-eosin. Fig. 3. Protuberated wall surface of a shrunken *C. bovis* bladder. Nuclei of subcuticullar cells accumulated at the base of the protuberances; beneath them strands of fibres(f) of the main muscles of the bladder wall. Very marked hairlike processes(e). Weigert-van Gieson (375×).

## Plate IV

Comparison of the bladder wall of *C. cellulosae* (right) and *C. bovis* (left) in total mounts. Fig. 1 and 2 focussed at the peaks of the wartlike formations and the protuberances. Fig. 3 and 4 focussed at the base of these formations. In *C. cellulosae* the nuclei of the subcuticular layer (Fig. 4) are evenly distributed, in *C. bovis* these cells are concentrated at the base of the protuberances (Fig. 3). In an expanded wall of *C. cellulosae* the subcuticular cell layer loses its character of evenly distributed nuclei (Fig. 6) while in *C. bovis* (Fig. 5) the nuclei are evenly arranged. Fig. 1,2 and 4,5 Weigert's ferric haematoxylin, Fig. 3 and 6 Jasvoin (330×).

## Plate V

Fig. 1. Section through the spiral canal of *C. cellulosae* showing the well arranged fibrous tissue on its surface (bottom left) constituting the surface of the invaginated portion where it faces the bladder cavity. This parenchyma of the folds of the invaginated canal, packed with calcareous corpuscles, is covered with a thick, dark cuticle. Haematoxylin-eosin. Fig. 2. In the section through the invaginated portion of *C. cellulosae* the calcareous corpuscles in the parenchyma are demonstrated with Kossa's method. (650×).

## Plate VI

Histological structures of the cerebral cysticercus. Fig. 1. The folds in the initial part of the entrance canal (100×). Fig. 2. The folds in the entrance canal (70×). Fig. 3. Longitudinal section through the invaginated portion (14×). Mallory's phosphotungstic haematoxylin. Fig. 4. Transverse section through the entrance canal (30×). Weigert-van Gieson. a — invaginated scolex; b — spiral canal; c — transition from the spiral canal to the entrance canal (d); e — loosely arranged tissue on the surface of the invaginated portion facing the bladder cavity; f — bladder wall; k — openings of the excretory canals.

## Plate VII

Fig. 1. Structures of the racemose cysticercus enclosed in the encapsulating tissue in the fissura interhaemisphaerica. The necrotic portion (left) is almost continuous with the bladder with its wartlike surface. In this section the expanded bladder (right) is separated by the encapsulating tissue (11×). Fig. 2. Bladder wall of a racemose cysticercus with a rim of hairlike projections on the folded surface and a dilated system of excretory canals in the parenchyma of the wall. Haematoxylin-eosin (300×).

## Plate VIII

Fig. 1. Necrotic focus with a cysticercus pressing into the intercerebral groove in the region of the septum pellucidum. Photograph. Fig. 2. Necrotic part of a racemose cysticercus in an inflammatory encapsulation at the base of the brain. Only the proliferating bud (a) of the bladder wall with a still undisturbed histological structure can be seen next to the a. basilaris. Haematoxylin-eosin (10×).

## Plate IX

Fig. 1. Solitary case of a strongly proliferating and branching, racemose cysticercus showing the successive formation of lumina in the solid protrusions. Fig. 2. Another completely necrotic portion of the same cysticercus enclosed in granulation tissue. Proliferating bladders only on its surface (bottom and right). (5×). Weigert van Gieson.

## Plate X

Typical bladders of the racemose cysticercus — material from an observation by Karpíšek and Valach (1952). Fig. 1. The section shows the irregular shape of the bladders (10×). Fig. 2. The histological structure of the wall of these bladders with a marked, wartlike surface. Haematoxylin-eosin (60×).

## Plate XI

Fig. 1. Outgrown scolex in the entrance canal of a *C. cellulosae* from the brain. Pits from the detached and fallen out hooks can be seen on the rostellum. Gomori (40×). Fig. 2. Outgrown scolex in the remnant of the entrance canal in a calcified, necrotic focus with hooks retained on the rostellum. The structure of the parasite is still visible because of unevenly distributed calcium deposition. Kossa (65×). Fig. 3. The neck with the outgrowing scolex in the invaginated canal of *C. bovis* sected out. Fig. 4. The same cysticercus after evagination showing the marked difference between the narrow, outgrowing portion with the scolex and the folded wall of the invaginated canal. Fig. 5. *C. crassiceps* with the outgrown scolex rising above the surface of the bladder. Photograph (7×).

## Plate XII

Fig. 1. Section of a *C. cellulosae* from the muscles of swine. Goldner (12×). Fig. 2. Evagination of the scolex of *C. cellulosae* inside the vestibule, middle stage of process. Weigert - van Gieson (25×).

## Plate XIII

Fig. 1. The lymphatic capillary in the skeletal muscles of swine dilated by the developing cysticercus. The bladder is growing round the parenchymatous portion. Connective tissue in the capillary wall is very dense (right). A similar density of connective tissue (left) in the muscles of the wall of another collapsed, lymphatic capillary with a slitlike lumen. Goldner (12×). Fig. 2. Extensive infestation of the brain of man. Cysticerci present in the cavities of the white matter in the region of the basal ganglia. Mallory's phosphotungstic haematoxylin (5,5×).

## Plate XIV

Fig. 1. A lymphatic capillary dilated by the fully developed *C. cellulosae* situated at the crossing points of the capillaries where connective tissue is thicker. At this site the tissue is less dilated than that of the thin-walled capillary and cuts into the bladder like a connective tissue septum. Fig. 2. Histological section through a capillary showing its dilatation by the parasite (bottom left). The section shows the twice interrupted course of the narrow, slitshaped lumen of this capillary occurring at the crossing points of the capillary network where connective tissue is thicker. Goldner (12×).

## Plate XV

Fig. 1. Interfascicular septum dilated by the fully developed *C. bovis* lying close to a thicker septum. Fig. 2. *C. bovis* in an advanced stage of resorption and development of the inflammatory encapsulation surrounded by necrotic exudate (6.5×). Fig. 3. Tangential section through the connective tissue capsule surrounding *C. bovis*. Its inner surface adjoining the bladder of the cysticercus forms marked layer of cells with nuclei arranged in parallel. The first infiltrated cells are found round the vessels of the encapsulating connective tissue (145×). Weigert - van Gieson.

## Plate XVI

Fig. 1 and 2. Histological proof of the identity of necrotic remnants of a cerebral cysticercus with Gomori's method. Fig. 1. The structure of the outgrown scolex and the bladder wall can be distinguished from the necrotic exudate (65×). Fig. 2. Degenerated, necrotic bladder wall permeated with fluid and still showing signs of the original division into a superficial cuticular layer and a lower parenchymatous portion (left) of hyaline appearance (160×). Fig. 3. The calcareous corpuscles in the calcified remnants of the cysticercus tissue differing greatly in shape and size from the grains of the calcium deposits. Fig. 4. Calcium deposits in the hyaline connective tissue encapsulation of the remants of the cysticercus containing only basophilic grains. Haematoxylin-eosin (580×). Fig. 5. The dilated canal system of the autolyzing bladder wall of the cysticercus contains a granular substance resembling a pigment. Mallory's phosphotungstic haematoxylin. This can be compared with the normal bladder wall shown in Fig. 6. Haematoxylin-eosin (130×).

## Plate XVII

Fig. 1. Protuberated wall surface of the collapsed bladder of *Coenurus cerebralis*. Nuclei of subcuticular cells accumulated at the base of the protuberances. Hairlike processes(c) on the surface of the cuticle are very low. Lacunae of the upper duct system very dilated. Weigert - van Gieson. Fig. 2. Wall of the racemose cyst of a cerebral cysticercus with a remarkably wartlike surface of its cuticle from an unexpanded, folded part of the cyst wall. The arrangement of subcuticular cells into a row is very regular, the canal system is in keeping with that of *C. cellulosae*. Haematoxylin-eosin (375×). Fig. 3. Surface of two proliferating buds of the racemose form of brain cysticercus with granulation tissue between them. The visible fibres of the subcuticular muscles are of the same size as those of *C. cellulosae*. Mallory's phosphotungstic haematoxylin (700×).

## Plate XVIII

Fig. 1 and 2. Parasitic formations in liver granulomas of man. Fig. 1. Necrotic, calcified exudate in the encapsulating, hyaline nodule; a spherical, parenchymatous formation measuring 180 μm in diameter was found in the middle of its hollow. Goldner (25×). Fig. 2. Structure of a young cysticercus with a differentiated surface layer and a central body cavity. Gomori. Fig. 3. *C. tenuicollis* in the highly infested liver of a lamb. Haematoxylin-eosin (22×). Fig. 4. Section through *C. tenuicollis* from the massively infested liver of a pig. Goldner (Fig. 2. and 4. 110×).

## Plate XIX

Fig. 1. A simple atrophy of the gray matter of the brain cortex caused by pressure of the adjoining cysticercus, but without further inflammatory changes. The cortex attenuated to one quarter of its original thickness. Mallory's trichrome (17×). Fig. 2. An almost complete discontinuity of the gray matter of the brain cortex in the groove under the shrivelled, necrotic and encapsulated cysticercus with an outgrown scolex extended to the bladder surface. Mallory's phosphotungstic haematoxylin (6×).

## Plate XX

Development of inflammatory changes round the degenerating cerebral cysticercus. Fig. 1. Origin of the infiltrate and multiplied fibroblasts in the layer adjoining the surface of the bladder. The parasite and the encapsulating tissue are so closely apposed that the boundary between them cannot be distinguished. Fig. 2. Proliferating fibroblasts and exudative cells on the surface of the already thickened fibrous encapsulation after the tearing away of the bladder wall. Fig. 3. Large accumulation of exudate consisting mainly of neutrophilic leukocytes between the bladder wall and the encapsulating tissue. Fig. 4. Giant cells formed on the surface of the connective tissue encapsulation after the shrinkage and necrosis of the parasite. Fig. 5. The necrotic portion of the bladder wall resorbed by giant cells. Fig. 6. Multiplied astroglial cells in a connective tissue glial scar. a — bladder wall; b — multiplying fibroblasts; c — brain tissue; k — necrotic exudate; f — fibrous connective tissue of the scar. Fig. 1—4 haematoxylin - eosin, Fig. 5 Goldner (120×), Fig. 6 Mallory's phosphotungstic haematoxylin (250×).

## Plate XXI

Fig. 1. Longitudinal section through the parenchymatous portion of *C. bovis* with a meandering, invaginated spiral canal on the bladder surface. Its opening is not on the section. The layer of well arranged connective tissue forming the lining of this portion opposite to the bladder cavity is seen. Fig. 2. Cross section through the parenchymatous portion of *C. bovis* with a particularly well marked layer of connective tissue on the surface. Inside it several sections of the spiral canal, the excretory canals and the sucker. Weigert - van Gieson (20×). Fig. 3. Transition of the thick cuticle of the invaginated canal of *C. bovis* into the surface of the bladder wall at its opening. Unlike the bladder wall the parenchyma of the canal is packed with calcareous corpuscles. Weigert — van Gieson. Fig. 4. Transition of the surface of the entrance canal of *C. bovis* into the surface of the bladder wall. The cuticle with the hairlike processes is uniformly high. A marked hypertrophy occurs in the basal layer of the entrance canal separating the more numerous subcuticular cells from the cuticle. No calcareous corpuscles are present in the parenchyma. Goldner (135×).

## Plate XXII

Fig. 1. Part of a young cysticercus in the muscle tissue of swine dilating the thin-walled lymphatic space. Top right — connective tissue supporting the bladder wall. The proliferating fold of the bladder wall grows round the parenchymatous portion of the larva with its complicated spiral canal. Goldner (30×). Fig. 2. Part of the wall of the proliferating fold of the bladder in Fig. 1. Most noticeable are the loops of the expanded subcuticular muscles under the cuticle; between them are compressed, subcuticular cells. Goldner (300×). Fig. 3. Subcuticular muscles in a partly autolyzed bladder wall of C. cellulosae coalesce into spherical formations; contrary to the main muscle fibres below, these stain the typical red of muscles. Goldner. Fig. 4. The wartlike surface of the bladder wall of *C. cellulosae* from the muscles of swine. The contracted muscles in the superficial formations are clearly visible (blue). Fig. 5. Expanded bladder wall of a cerebral cysticercus; in it the expanded subcuticular muscle groups of typical size. Mallory's phosphotungstic haematoxylin (350×).

## Plate XXIII

Fig. 1. The surface of the invaginated canal of *C. cellulosae* covered with a thick and probably very compressed cuticle causing the secondary folding of this wall; in it the characteristic deep grooves. Also the basal layer (pale stripe) under the cuticle is greatly thickened under the folds of the cuticle, but almost invisible under the grooves. The sections through the muscle fibres of both main layers, loose subcuticular cells and the parenchyma with calcareous corpuscles are also visible under the cuticle. Haematoxylin-eosin. Fig. 2. A thin, highly reactive layer on the surface of the cuticle of Fig. 1 becomes visible after staining with colloidal iron after Mowry (350×). Fig. 3. Tangential section through the surface of the invaginated canal from Fig. 1 showing the subcuticular network of muscle fibres crossed at right angles. Mallory's phosphotungstic haematoxylin. Fig. 4. The same tangential section as in Fig. 3. Impregnation with Gomori's method demonstrates the basal layer of the cuticle and in it the apertures for the cytoplasmatic extensions connecting the distal and perinuclear cytoplasm (350×). Fig. 5. A cerebral cysticercus with a differentiating entrance canal (top.). The most intensive staining occurs in the cuticle of the communicating part. Typical grooves (bottom) are seen in the cuticle of the spiral canal. A reconstruction of this cysticercus is in Fig. 16 left. Giemsa (30×).

## Plate XXIV

Fig. 1. Proliferating buds of the racemose cysticercus with a developing lumen. Between the buds is necrotic, inflammatory tissue. Giemsa (32×). Fig. 2. Surface of the proliferating bud from Fig. 1. The groups of expanded muscle fibres under the cuticle are typical of *C. cellulosae*. No calcareous corpuscles in the parenchyma. Mallory's phosphotungstic haematoxylin (350×). Fig. 3. Live *C. bovis* in the muscle; its wall is transparent at both ends but thickened in the centre because of a greater accumulation of connective tissue. The outlining muscle bundles were taken out to demonstrate the direct communication between the envelope of the cysticercus and the interfascicular septa of the fibrous connective tissue. Fresh material (3×). Fig. 4. Half of the cysticercus protruding from the surface of the cut through the muscle, showing the communication of the formation with the system of thicker tissue septa of a higher order. Only the peak of the formation is translucent, while its remaining parts are thickened by an accumulation of connective tissue containing clearly visible vessels filled with blood. Inflammatory changes and necrotic exudate inside the cyst are responsible for the yellow colour of its tip. Fresh material (3×).

## Plate XXV

Fig. 1. *C. cellulosae* parenchymatous portion with an invaginated canal with a very folded wall. At its end the terminal zone of growth is noteworthy for the accumulation of nuclei (blue). Giemsa (30×). Fig. 2. Zone of growth beneath the sucker (top) after the evagination of the scolex originating from an accumulation of marked, subcuticular cells. No calcareous corpuscles in the parenchyma. Haematoxylin-eosin (150×). Fig. 3. Outgrown scolex in the opening of the spiral canal of *C. cellulosae*. Fig. 4. Another section through the parenchymatous portion of Fig. 3. One section through the spiral canal shows the outgrown neck in cross section, the other shows the neck receding from the wall of the spiral canal. Haematoxylin-eosin (35×). Fig. 5. Cysticercus in the cerebellar cortex under the meninges; its growth and pressure disturbs greatly the cerebellar gyrus. Haematoxylin-eosin (15×).

## Plate XXVI

Fig. 1. Giant cells phagocytozing part of the bladder wall (red) in the necrotic exudate of the cerebral cyst. Goldner (160×). Fig. 2. Necrotic outgrown scolex of a cerebral cysticercus. The rostellar hooks stained selectively blue with Giemsa (50×). Fig. 3. Shrivelled, subependymal scar after the collapse of the cavity from which the cysticercus escaped. Goldner (12×). Fig. 4. Scars in the basal ganglia of the brain with remnants of the exudate in the centre. The hooks found in the hyaline tissue confirmed that these scars originated from a cysticercus (12×). Fig. 5. Hooks of a cysticercus in the hyaline connective tissue of a minute scar at the base of the brain (40×). Weigert - van Gieson.

All figures in the plates are original photomicrographs made by the author.

PLATE I

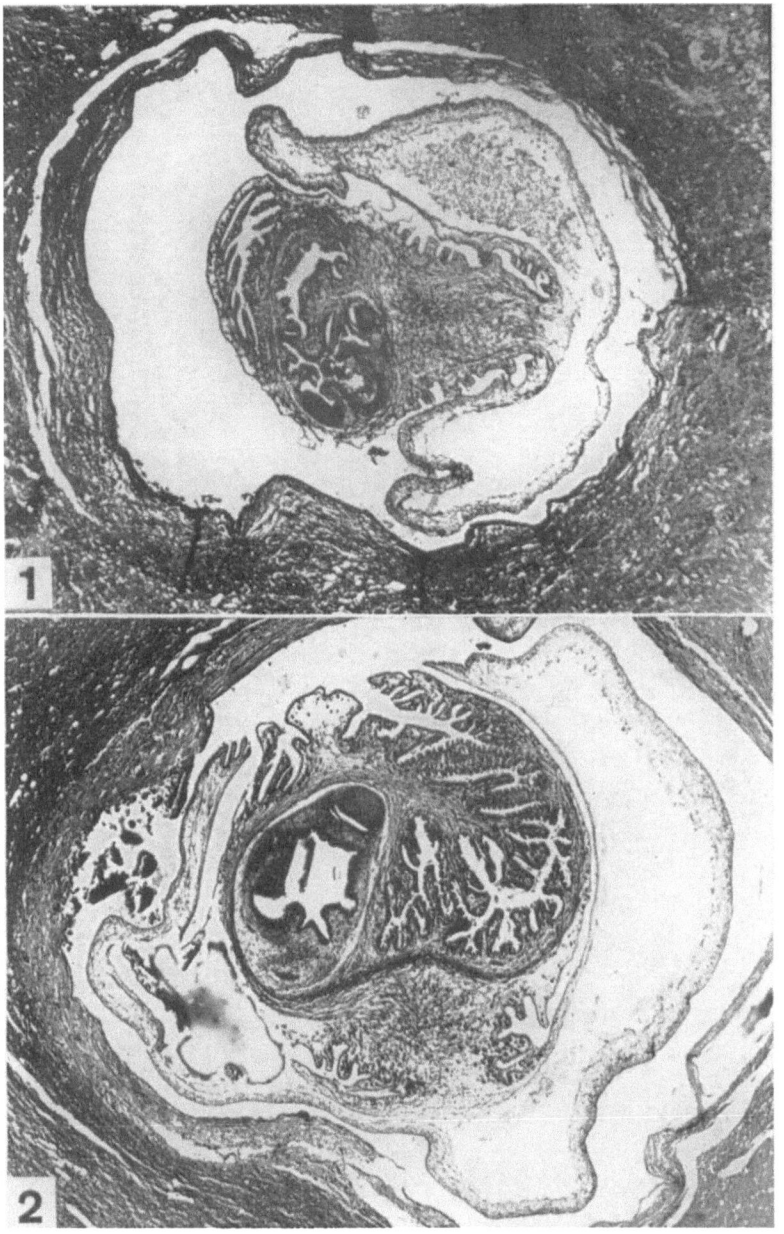

PLATE II

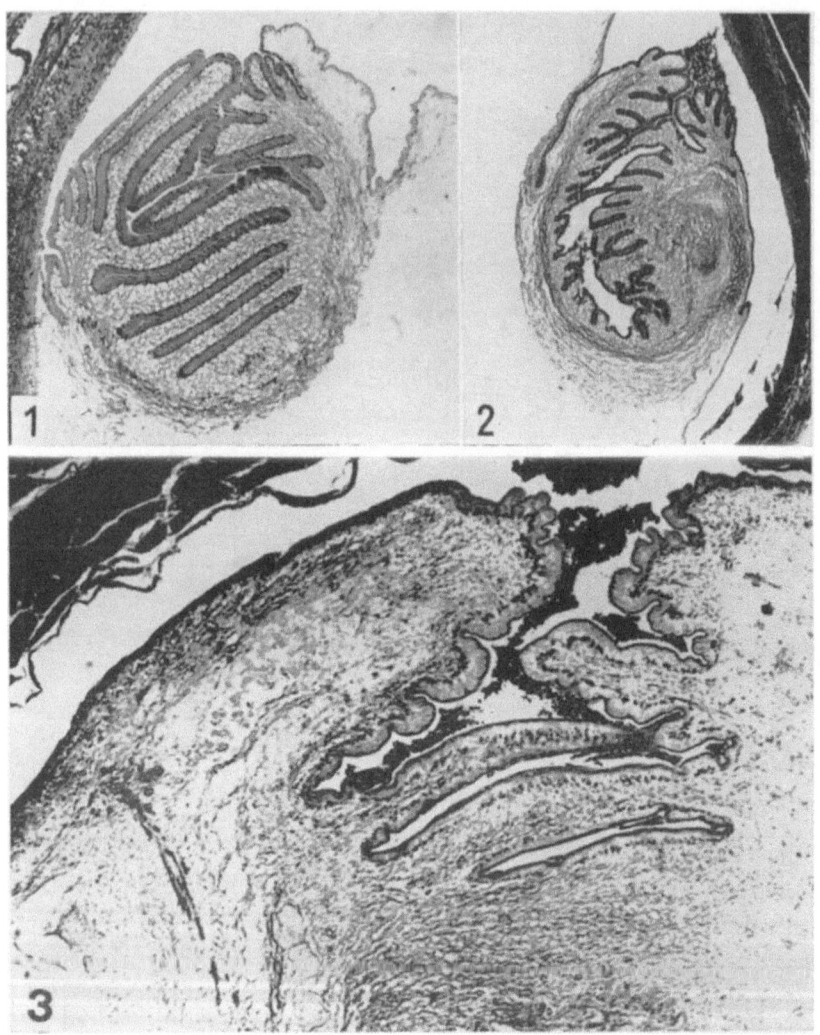

PLATE III

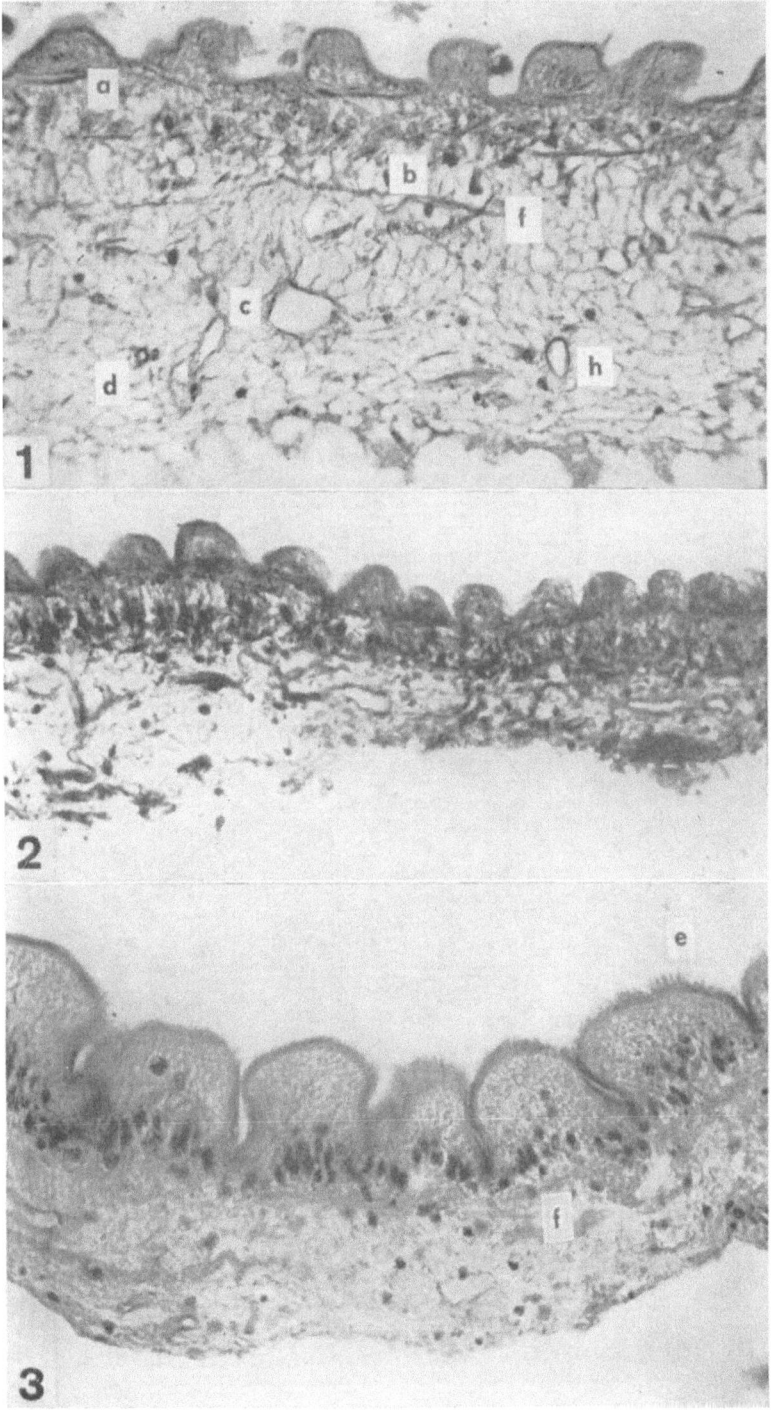

PLATE IV

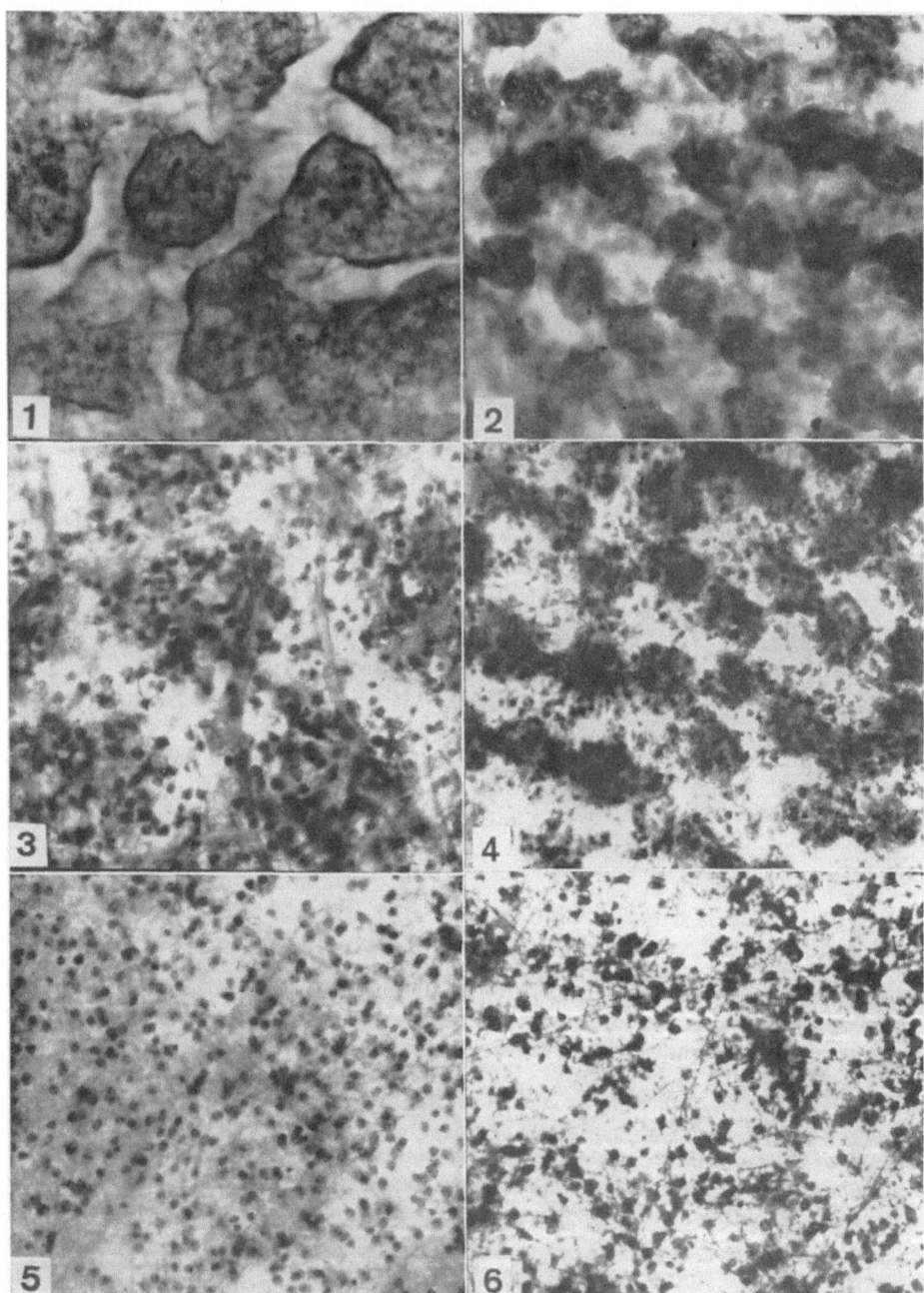

PLATE V

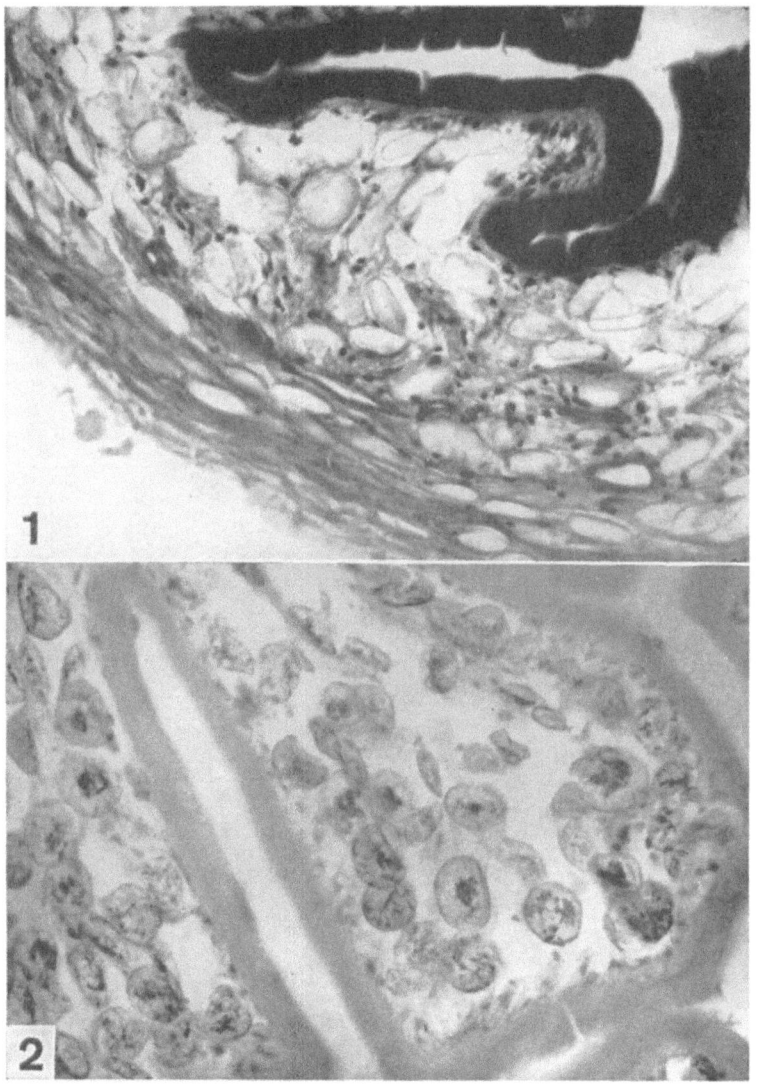

PLATE VI

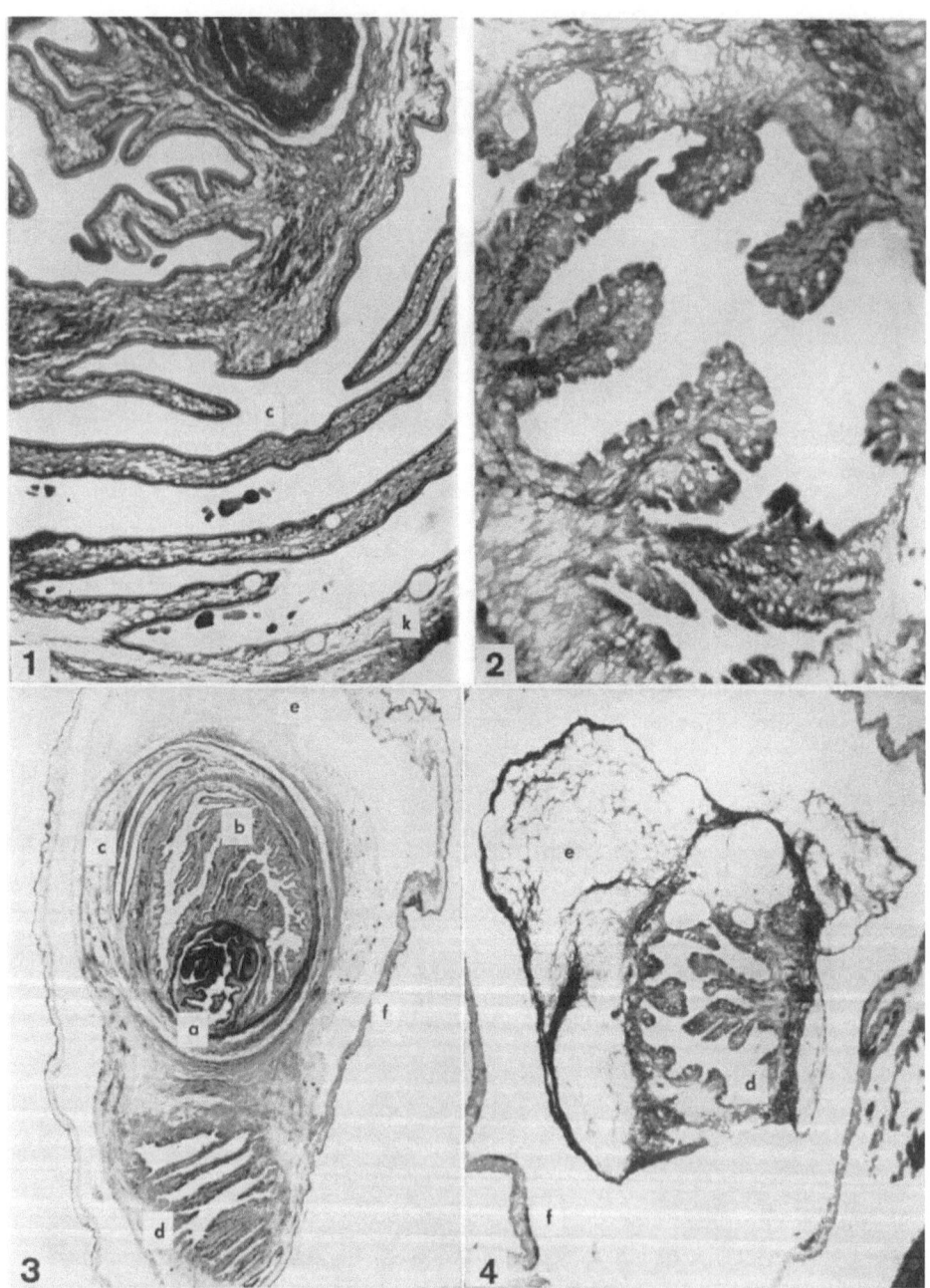

PLATE VII

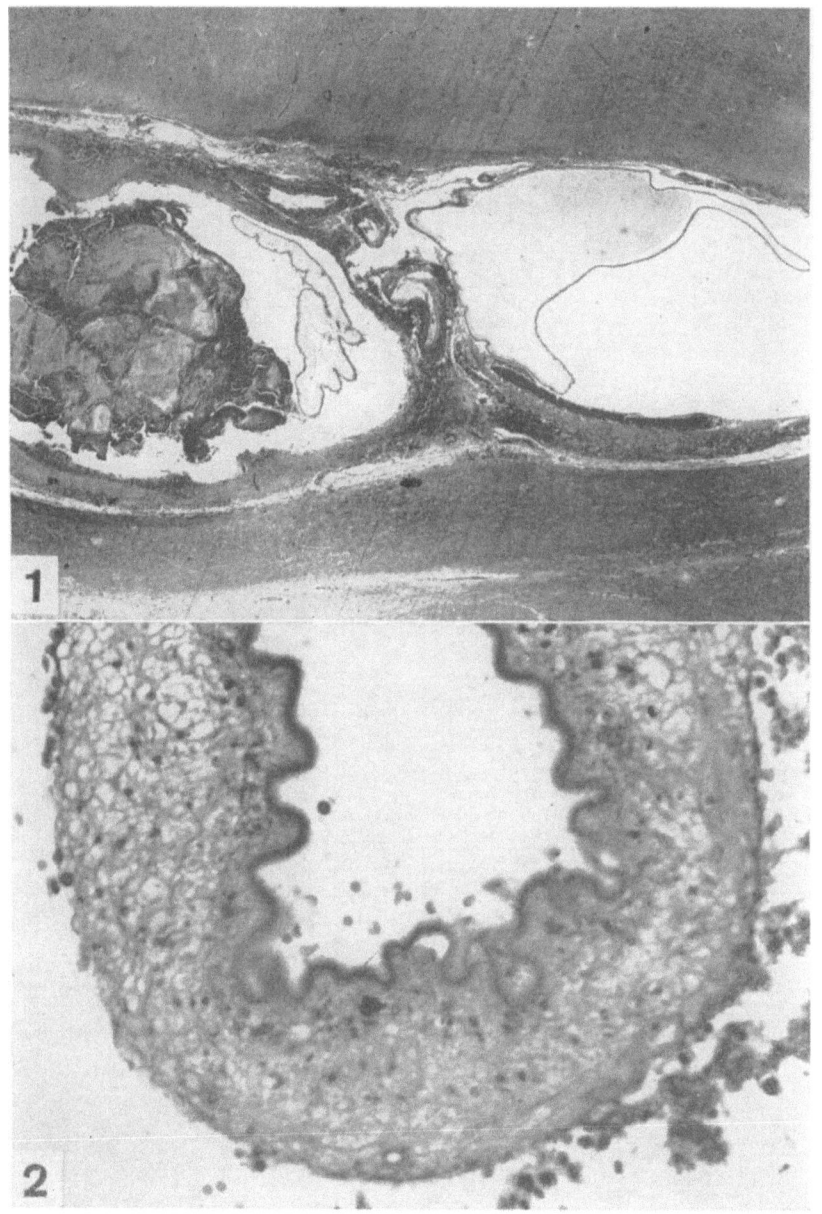

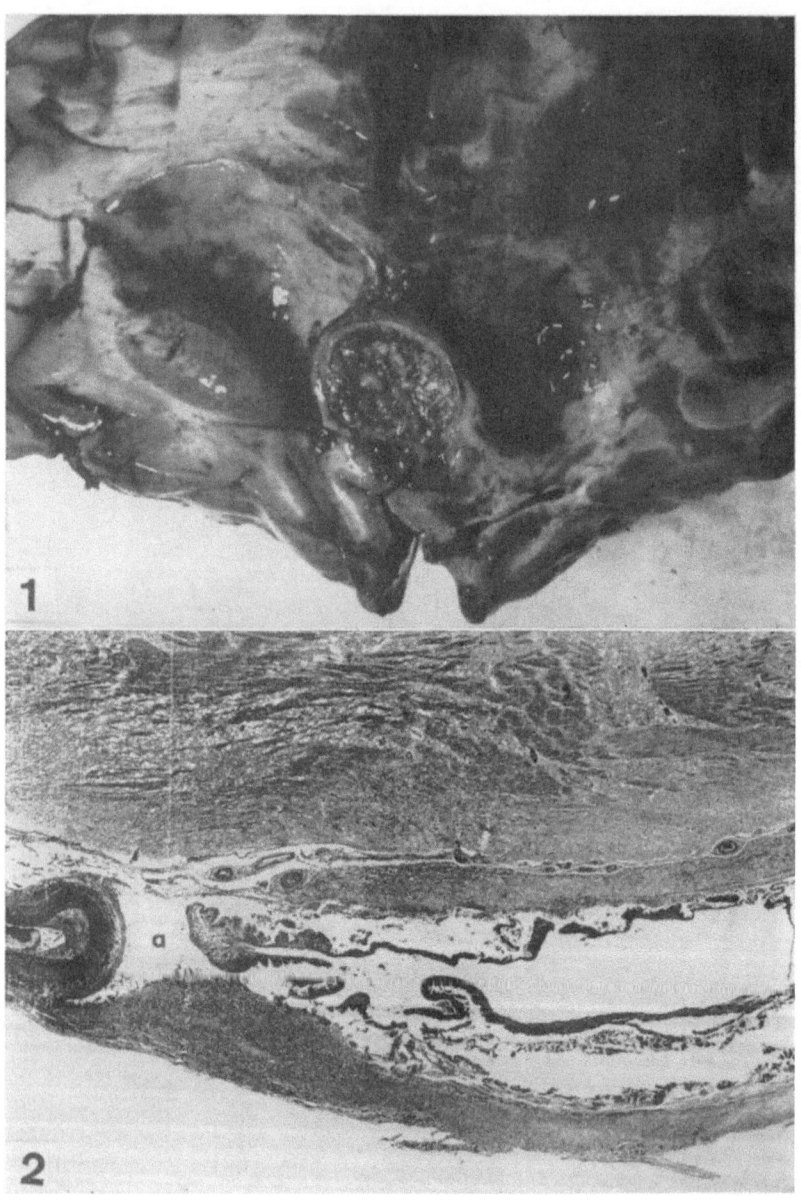

PLATE VIII

PLATE IX

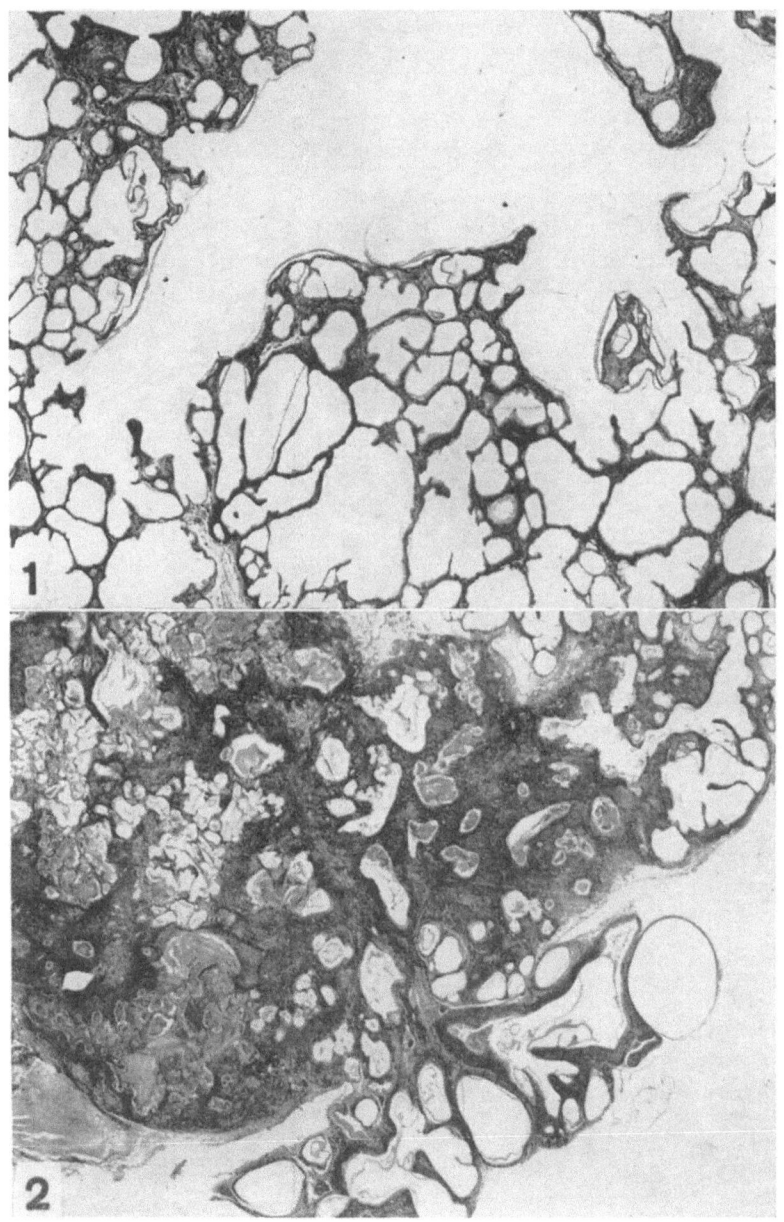

PLATE X

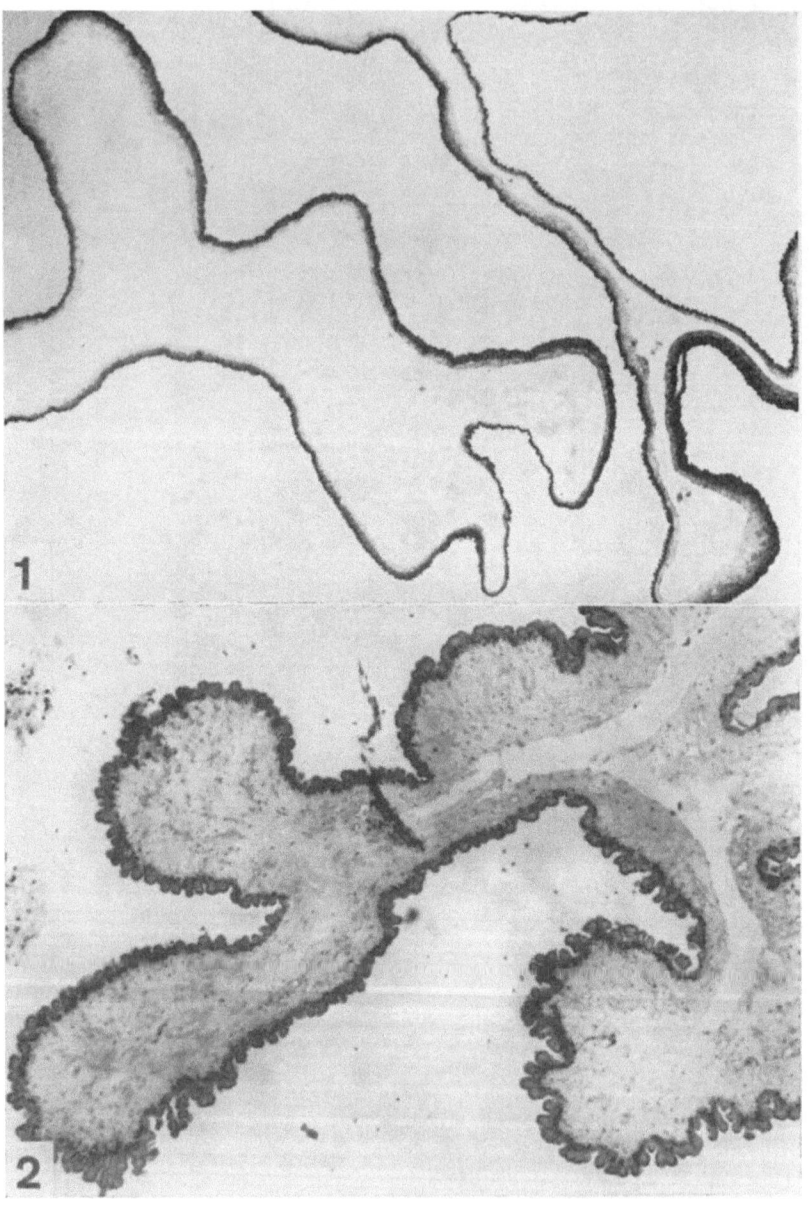

PLATE XI

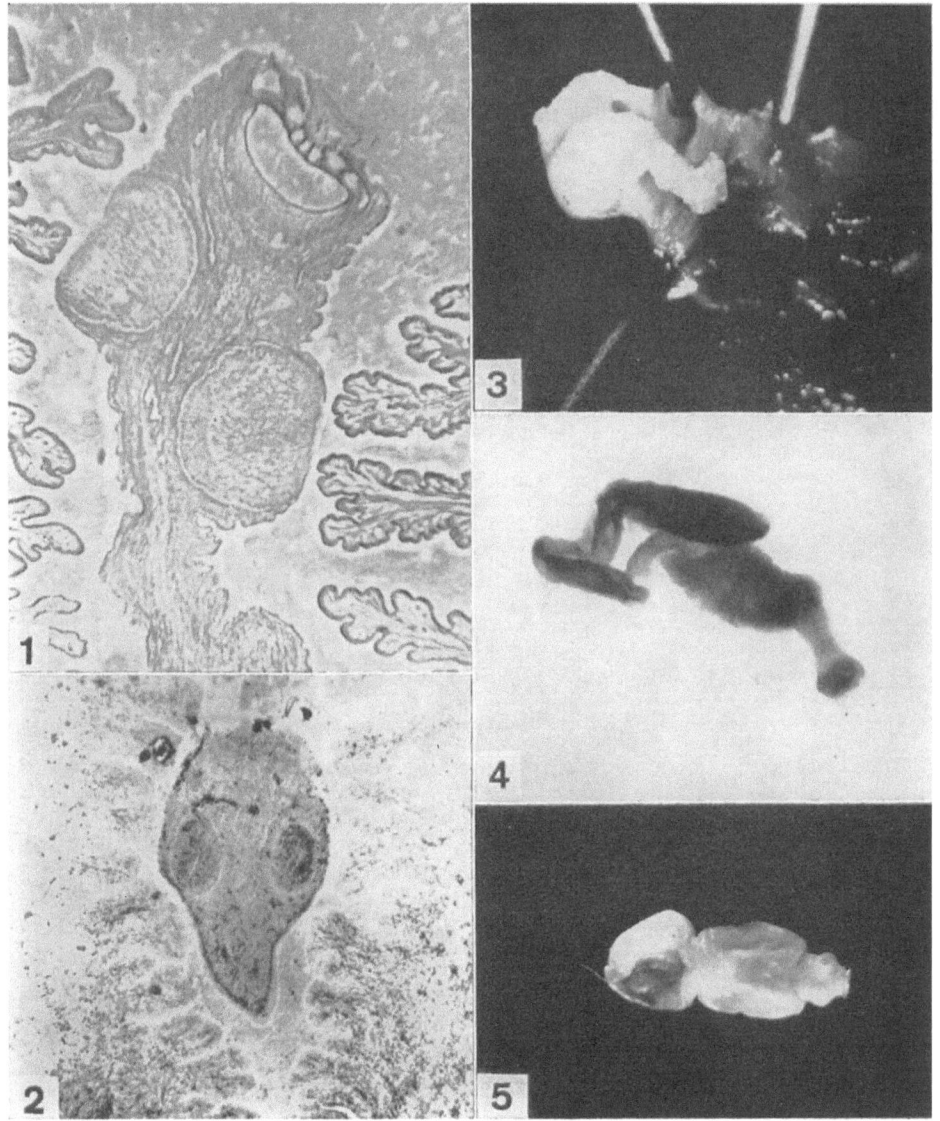

PLATE XII

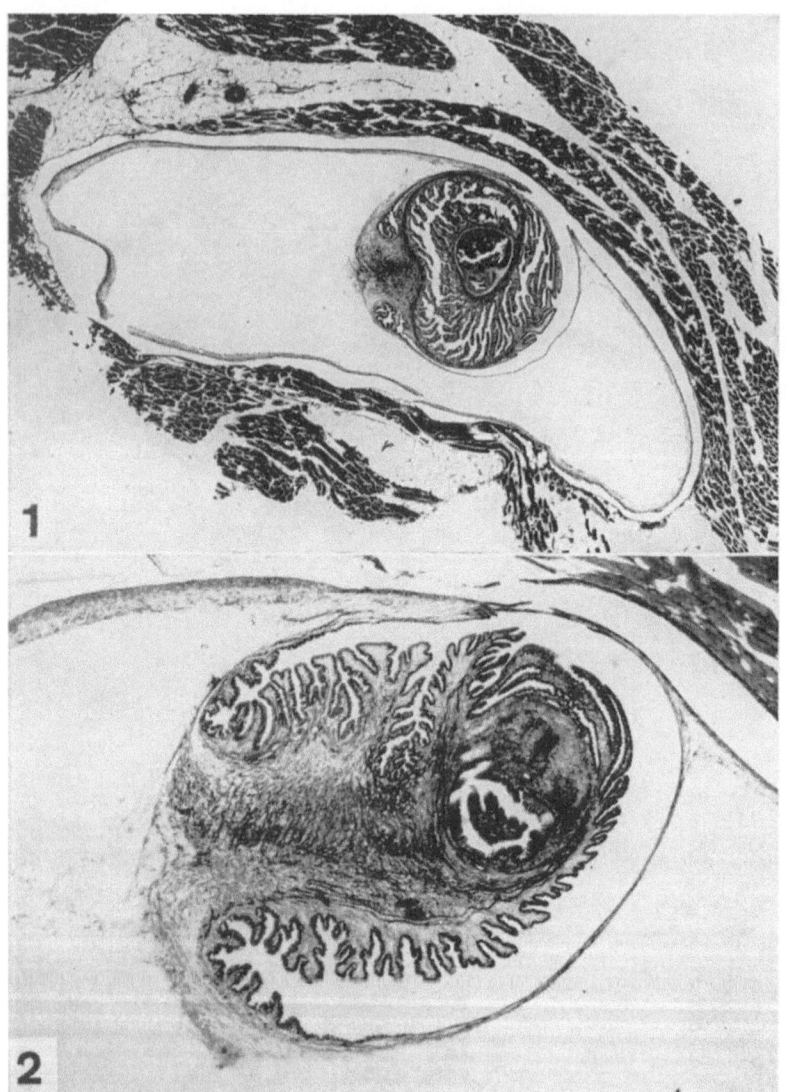

PLATE XIII

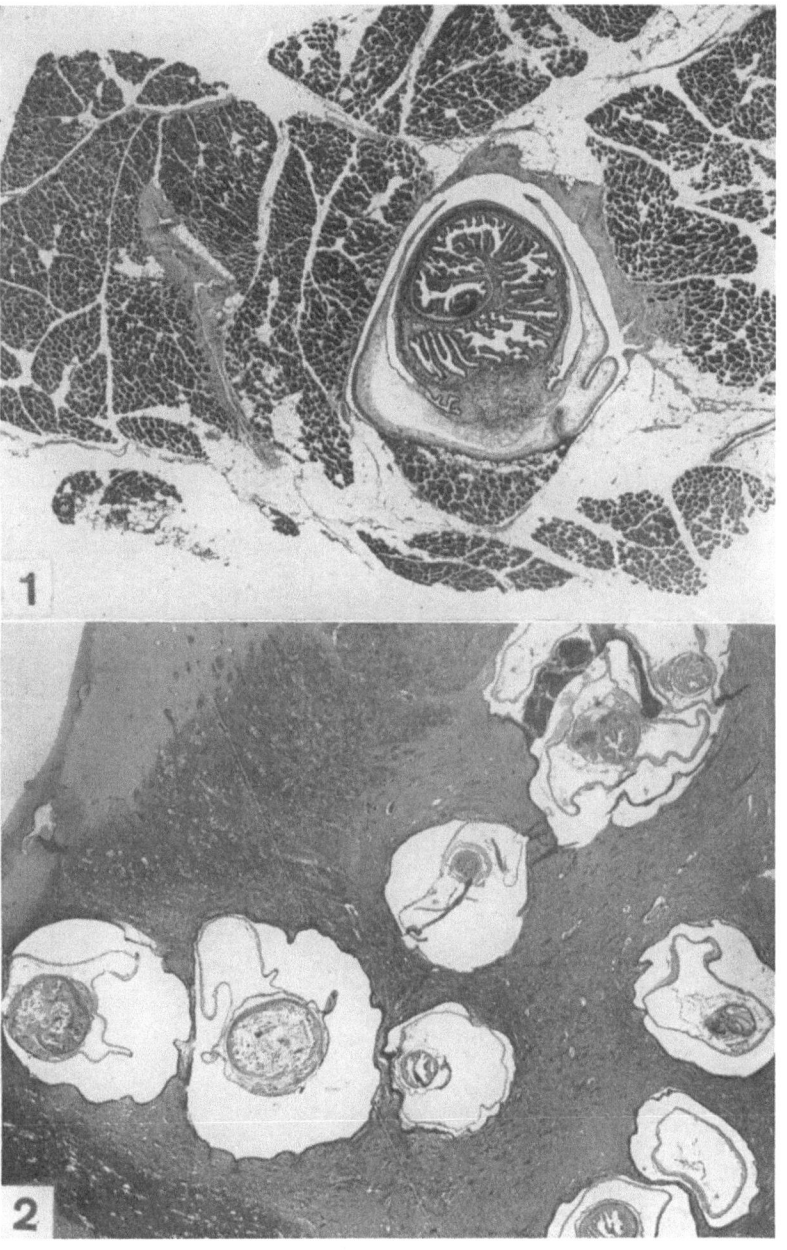

PLATE XIV

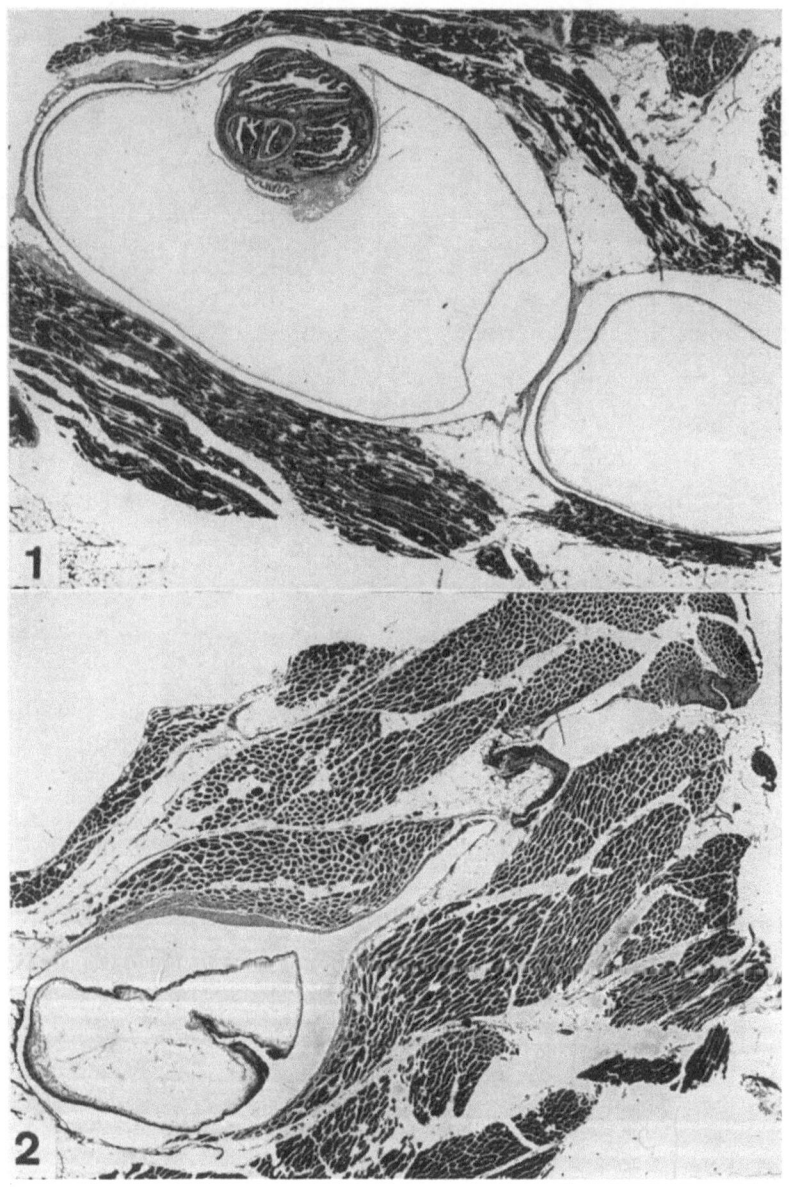

PLATE XV

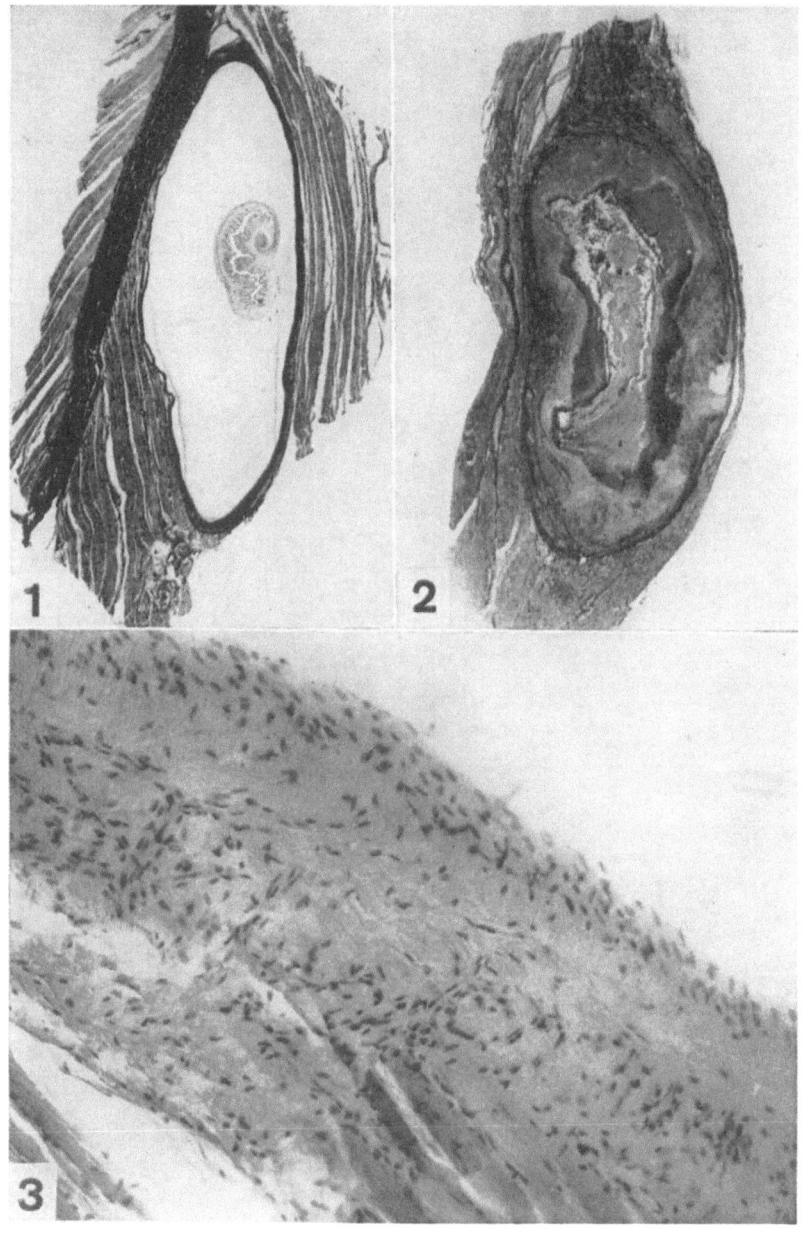

PLATE XVI

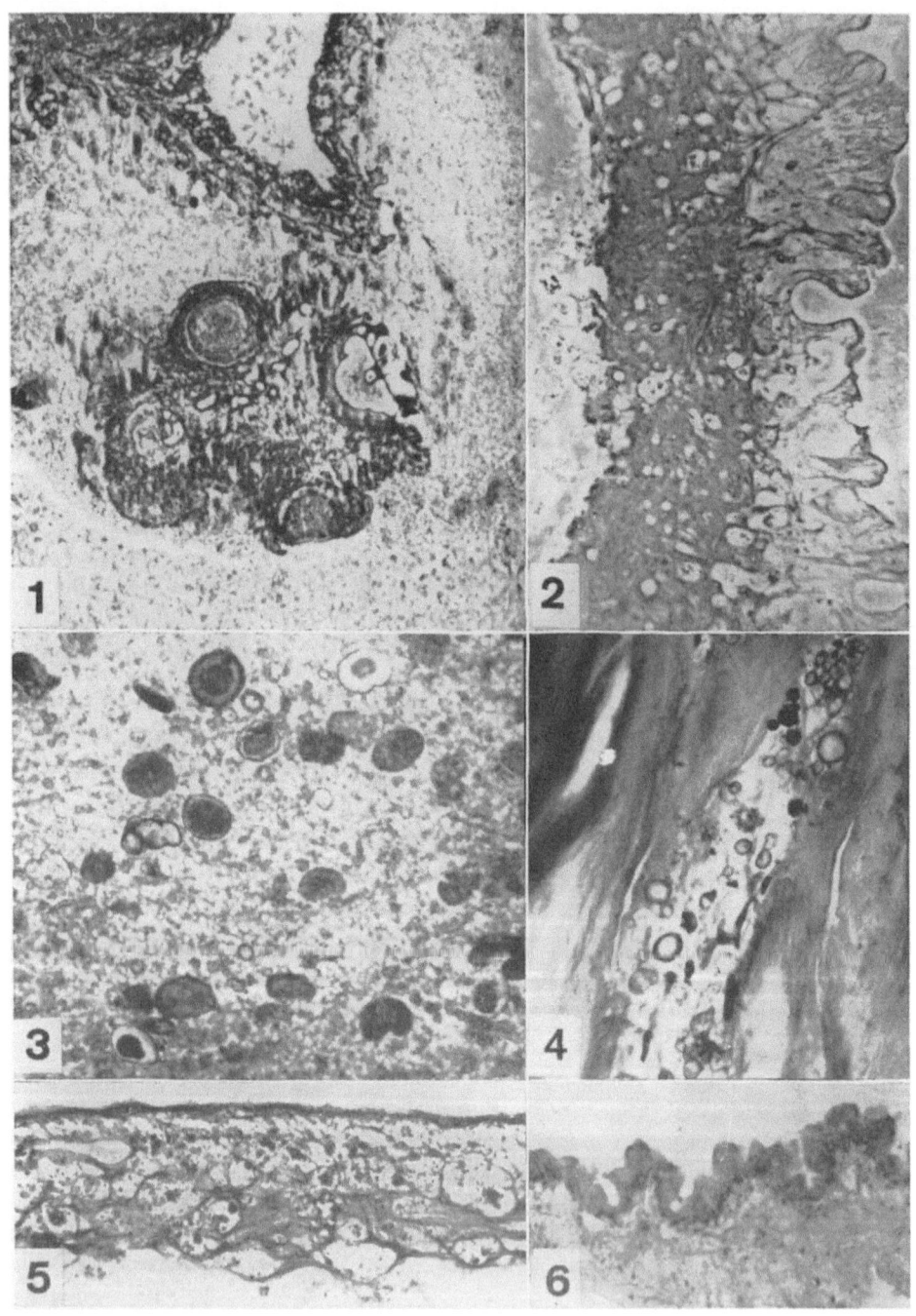

PLATE XVII

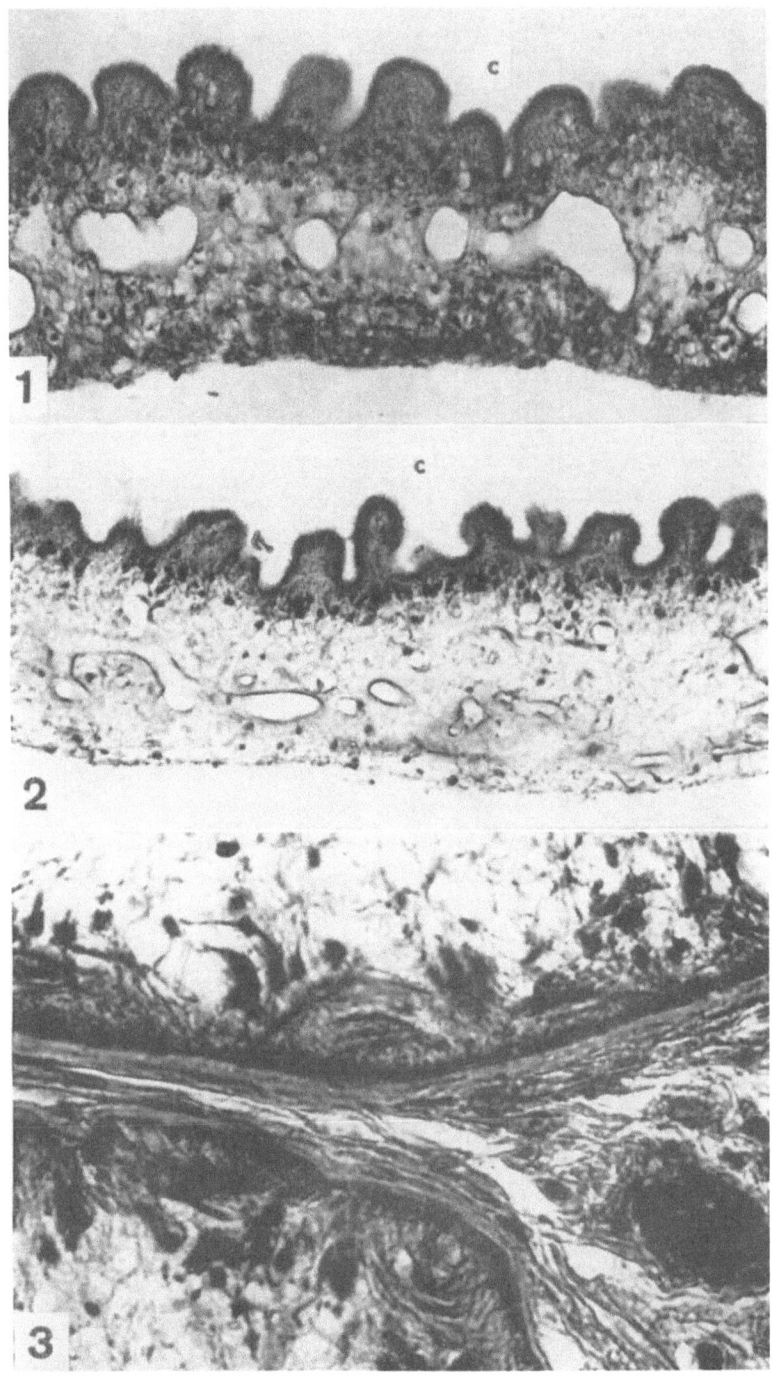

PLATE XVIII

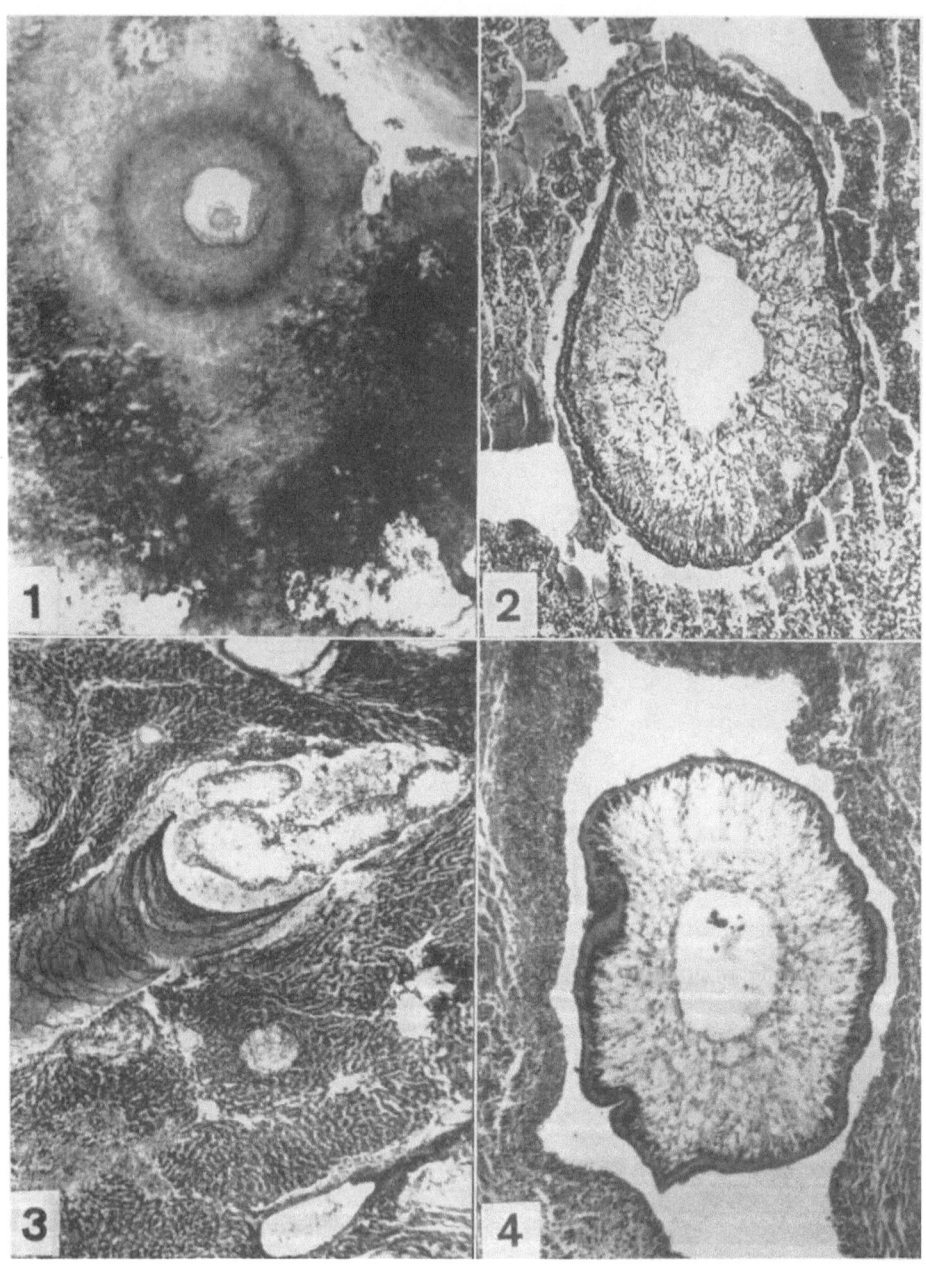

PLATE XIX

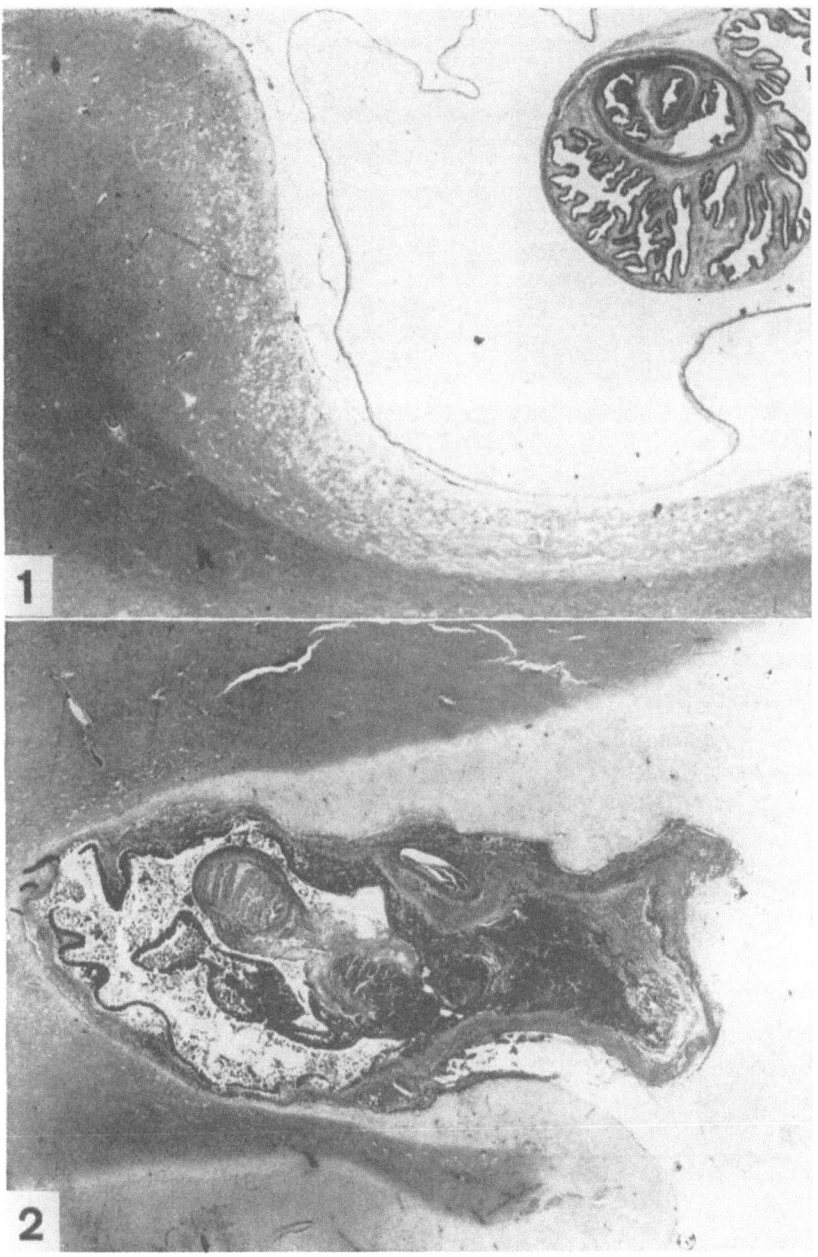

PLATE XX

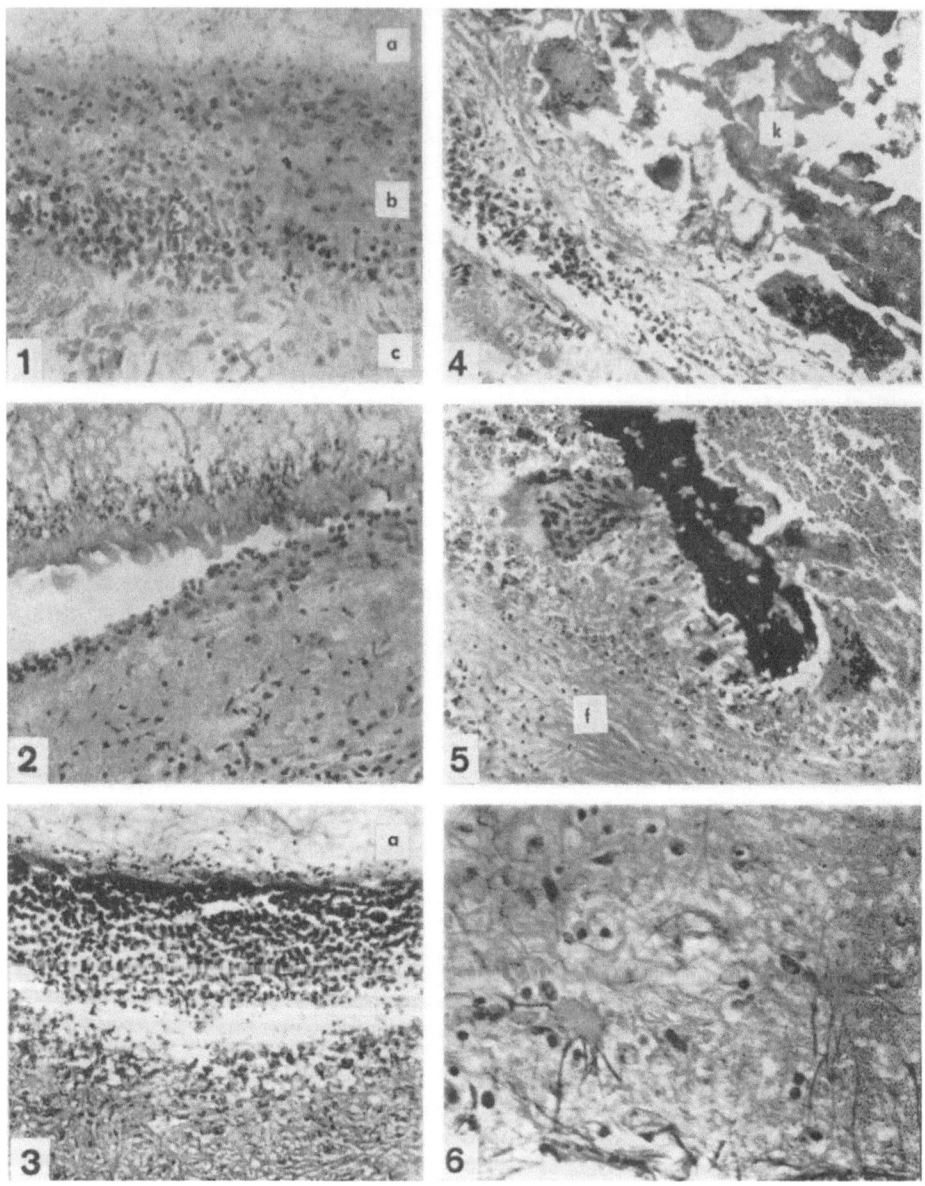

PLATE XXI

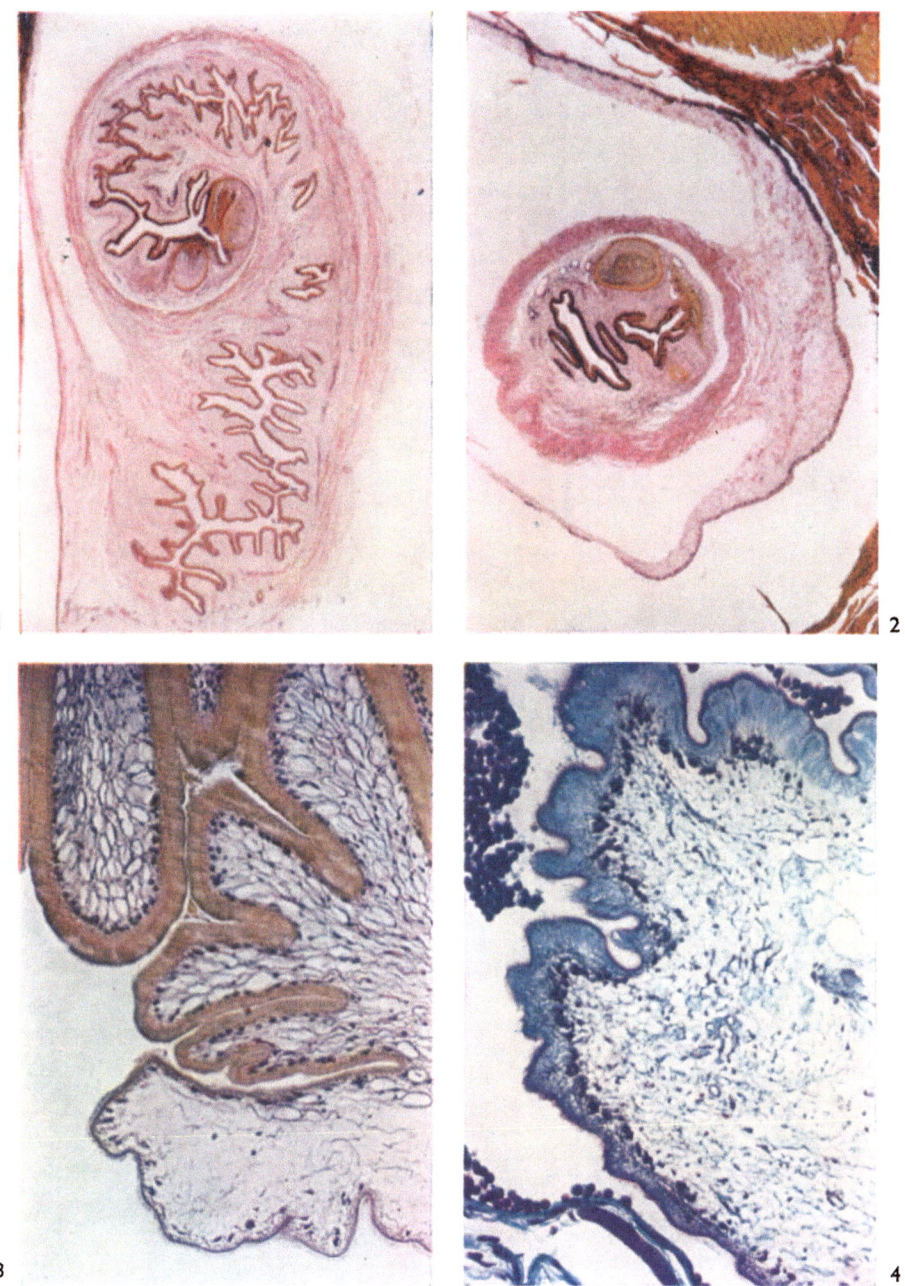

PLATE XXII

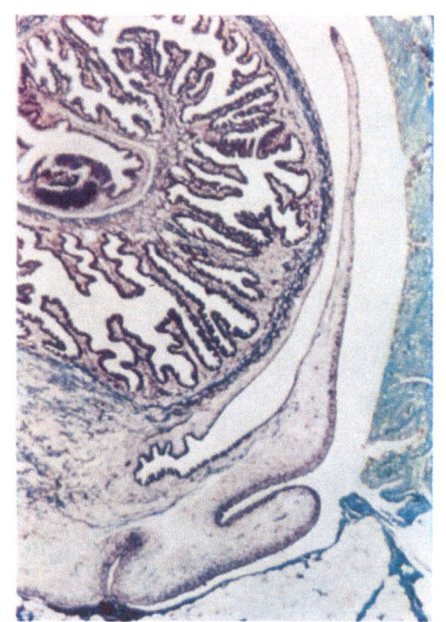
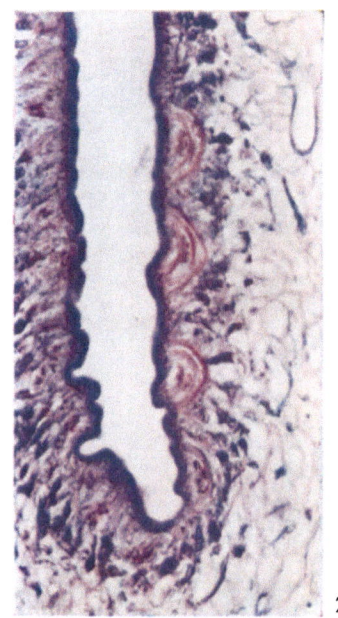

1

2

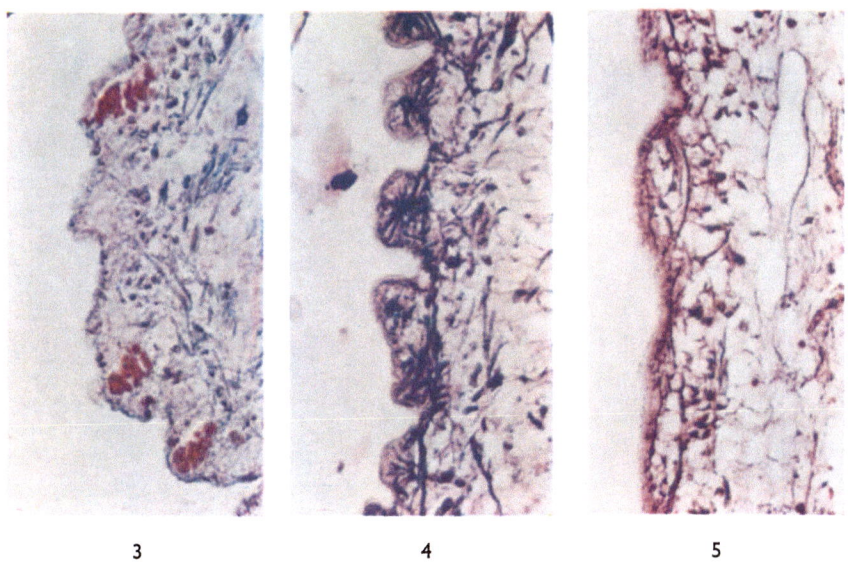

3

4

5

PLATE XXIII

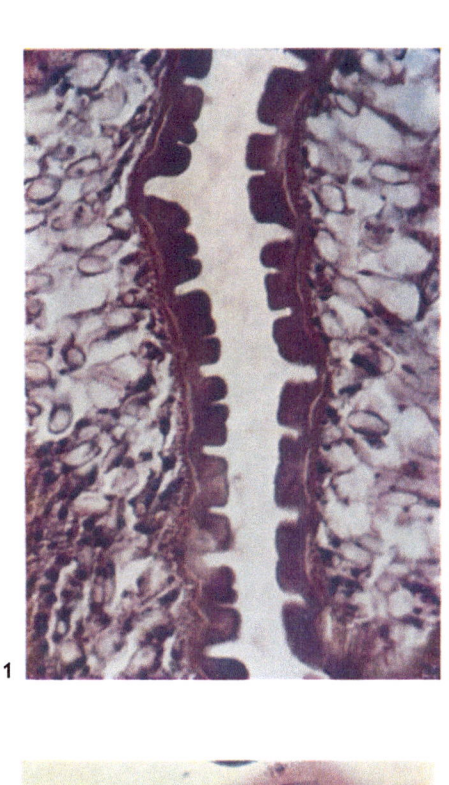

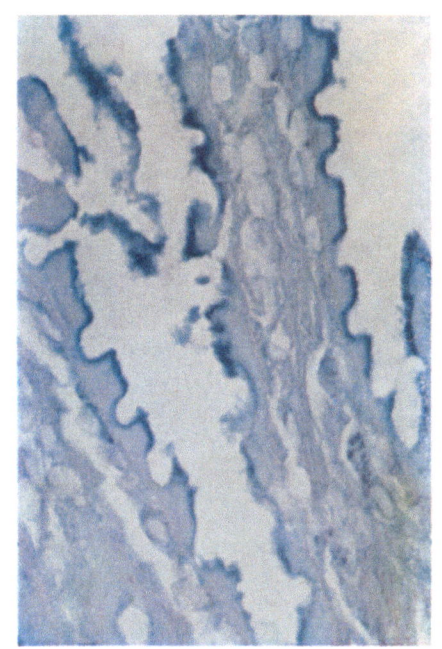

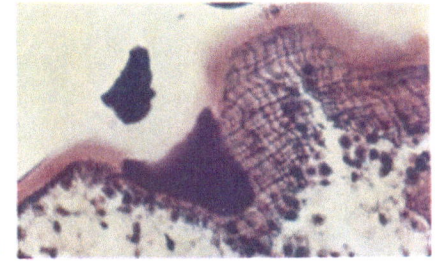

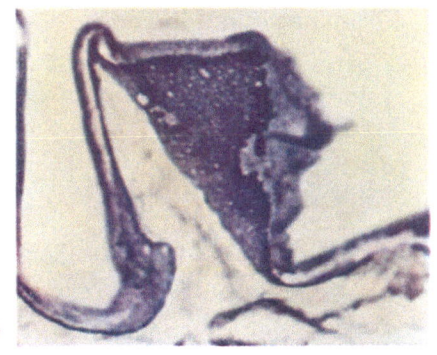

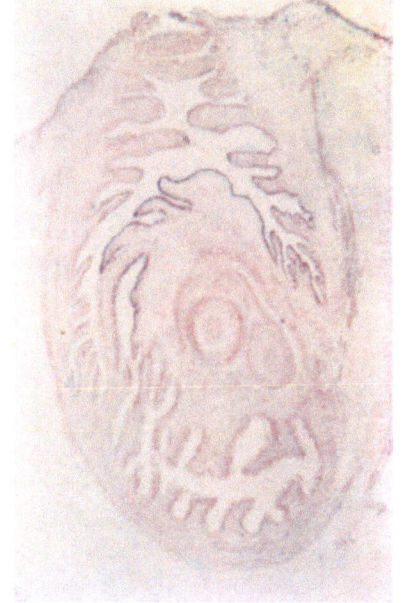

PLATE XXIV

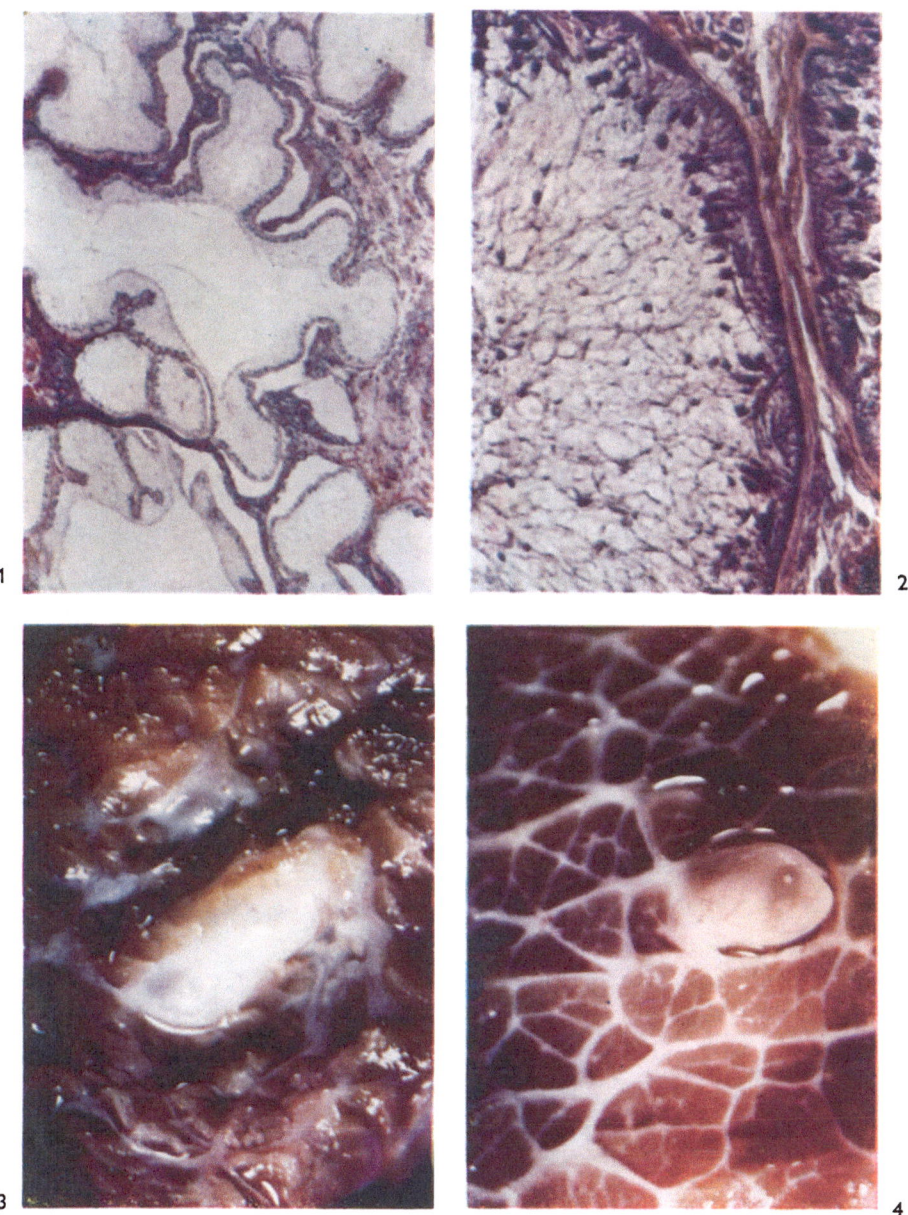

PLATE XXV

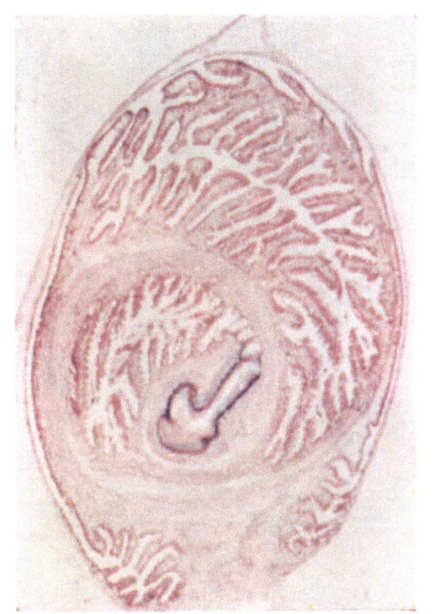

1

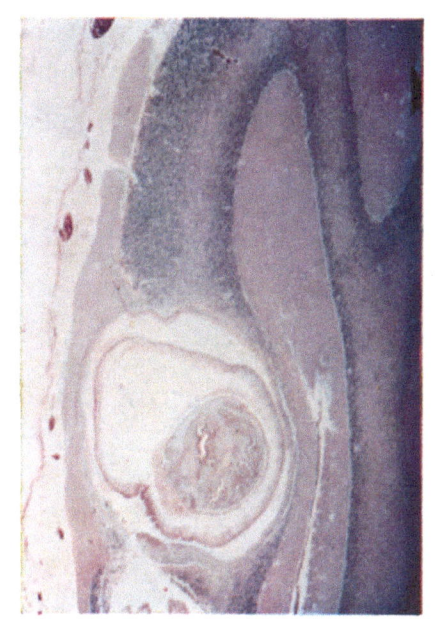

5

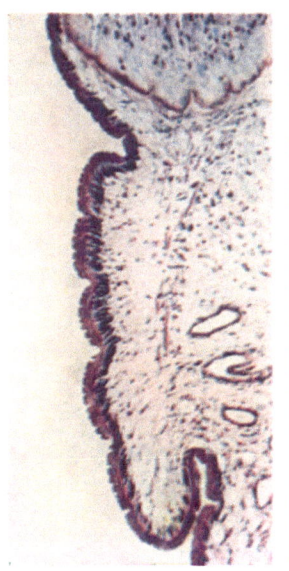

2

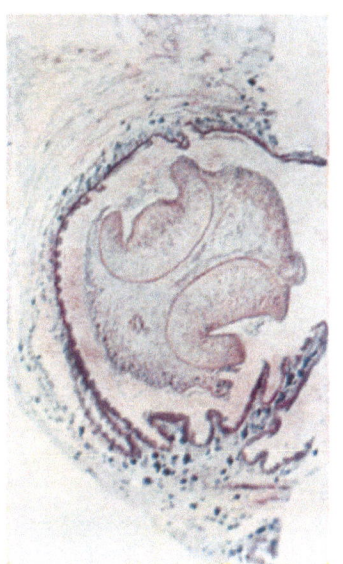

3

4

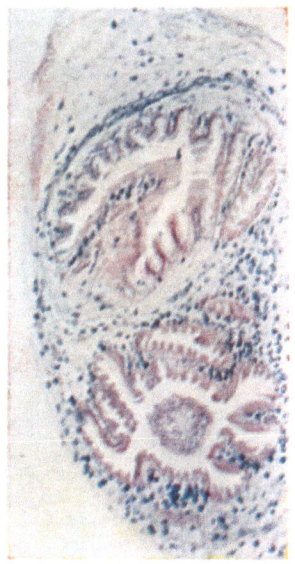

PLATE XXVI

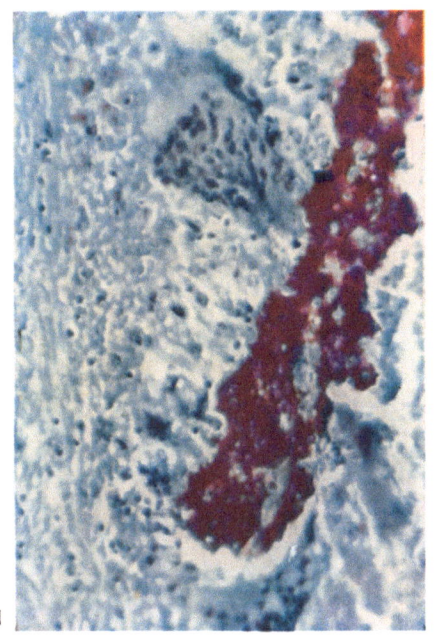

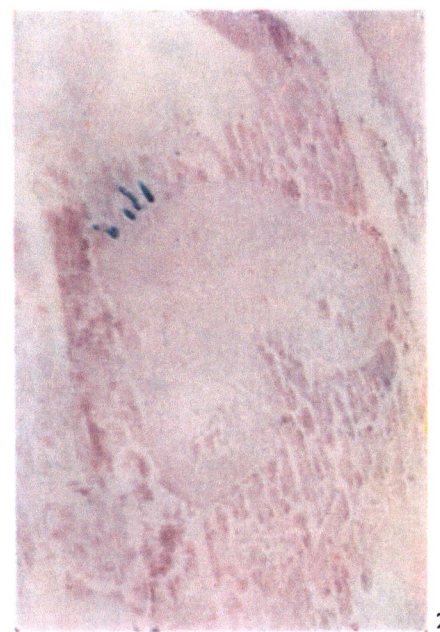

1

2

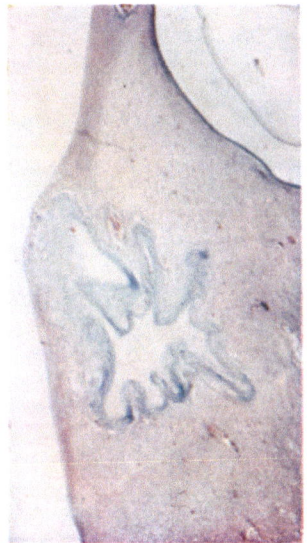

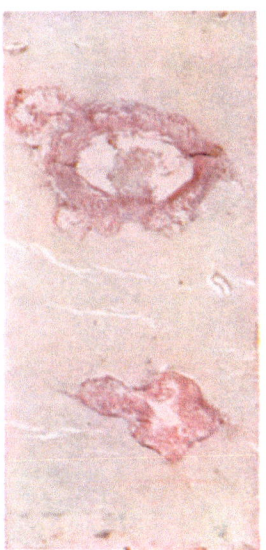

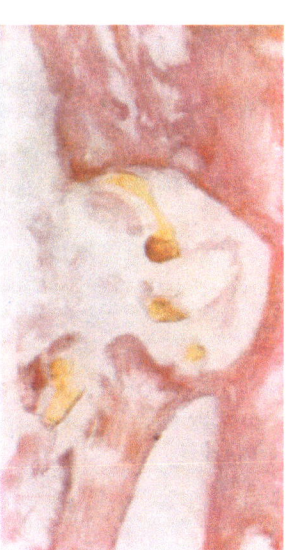

3

4

5